Scientific Researches in Health Sciences

Fatma Eti Aslan (ed.)

Scientific Researches in Health Sciences

PETER LANG

**Bibliographic Information published by the
Deutsche Nationalbibliothek**

The Deutsche Nationalbibliothek lists this publication in the Deutsche Nationalbibliografie; detailed bibliographic data is available online at http://dnb.d-nb.de.

Library of Congress Cataloging-in-Publication Data

A CIP catalog record for this book has been applied for at the Library of Congress.

The chapters in this book are first reviewed by the independent reviewers and then proof-read and edited by the editor. The opinions and views expressed in the articles are not necessarily those of the editor. All the views expressed in the book are purely that of the authors themselves and may not in any circumstances be regarded as stating an official position of Bahçeşehir University nor that of the editor of the book.

ISBN 978-3-631-79216-2 (Print)
E-ISBN 978-3-631-80264-9 (E-PDF)
E-ISBN 978-3-631-80265-6 (EPUB)
E-ISBN 978-3-631-80266-3 (MOBI)
DOI 10.3726/b16162

© Peter Lang GmbH
Internationaler Verlag der Wissenschaften
Berlin 2019
All rights reserved.

Peter Lang – Berlin · Bern · Bruxelles · New York · Oxford · Warszawa · Wien

This publication has been peer reviewed.

www.peterlang.com

Foreword

The increased knowledge in health care and the development of health-care technologies is a great contribution to scientific studies in this field.In this context, this book will contribute to the development of health sciences and the quality of patient care, with a total of 14 scientific original research articles of which eight are on physiotherapy and rehabilitation, five on nursing, and one on health management

A total of 29 researchers/writers who contributed to these scientific research articles prepared meticulously with great labor, and also contributed in the selection of articles and the preparation of the book for publication. I would like to thank Hayat Yalın, Hasan Kerem Alptekin, İshak Aydemir for their contributions to the health sciences and Fadime Çınar for editorial support.

Editor Prof. Dr. Fatma Eti Aslan

Contents

List of Contributors

Bülent Aksoy
Bahçeşehir University Health
Sciences Faculty, Physiotherapy
and Rehabilitation Department,
Istanbul, Turkey

Hasan Kerem Alptekin
Bahçesehir University, Faculty of
Health Sciences, Department of
Physiotherapy and Rehabilitation,
Istanbul, Turkey

Esra Atılgan
İstanbul Medipol University, Faculty
of Health Sciences, Physical Therapy
and Rehabilitation, Istanbul, Turkey

Leyla Ataş Balcı
Bahcesehir University, Faculty of
Health Sciences, Department of
Physiotherapy and Rehabilitation,
Istanbul, Turkey

Semra Bülbüloğlu
Department of Neonatal Intensive
Care Unit, Dr. Behcet Uz Child and
their Surgery Education and Research
Hospital, Izmir, Turkey

Fadime Çınar
Sabahattin Zaim University, Faculty of
Health Sciences, Health Management,
Istanbul, Turkey

Çiçek Duman
Bahcesehir University, Faculty of
Health Sciences, Physiotherapy and
Rehabilitation, Istanbul, Turkey

Fatma Eti Aslan
Department of Surgical Nursing,
Health Sciences Faculty, Bahcesehir
University, Istanbul, Turkey

Lütfü Hanoğlu
Istanbul Medipol University,
Faculty of Medicine, Department of
Neurology, Istanbul, Turkey

H. Serap İnal
Bahcesehir University, Faculty of
Health Sciences, Physiotherapy and
Rehabilitation, Istanbul, Turkey

Halim İşsever
Istanbul University Istanbul Medical
Faculty Public Health Department,
Istanbul, Turkey

Dilber Karagözoğlu Coskunsu
Bahcesehir University, Faculty of
Health Sciences, Physiotherapy and
Rehabilitation, Istanbul, Turkey

Evin Korkmaz Turkurka
Bahcesehir University, Institute
of Health Sciences Department of
Nursing, Istanbul, Turkey

Banu Kuran
Şişli Hamidiye Etfal Research and
Education Hospital, Istanbul,
Turkey

Gökay Kurtulan
Bahçeşehir University, Faculty of
Health Science, Health Management
Department, Istanbul, Turkey

Hazal Öksüz
Bahcesehir University, Faculty of
Health Sciences, Department of
Physiotherapy and Rehabilitation,
Istanbul, Turkey

Jülide Öncü Alptekin
Health Sciences University, Şişli
Hamidiye Education and Research
Hospital, Istanbul, Turkey

Emel Ece Özcan Ekşi
Bahçeşehir University Faculty
of Medicine, Physical Medicine
and Rehabilitation Department,
Istanbul, Turkey

Emel Özcan
İstanbul University Istanbul
Faculty of Medicine Department
of Physical Medicine and
Rehabilitation Deparment,
Istanbul, Turkey

Necmiye Sabuncu
Haliç University School of Nursing,
Istanbul, Turkey

Caferi Tayyar Selcuk
Dicle University, Medical Faculty,
Department of Plastic, Reconstructive
and Aesthetic Surgery and Burn
Center, Diyarbakır,Turkey

Ömer Şevgin
Beşiktaş Municipality, Directorate of
Health Affairs, Istanbul, Turkey

Feryal Subaşi
Yeditepe University, Faculty of
Health Sciences, Physiotherapy and
Rehabilitation, Istanbul, Turkey

Bahar Teksöz
Istanbul Physical Medicine and
Rehabilitation Education and
Research Hospital, Physical Medicine
and Rehabilitation Department,
Istanbul, Turkey

Gonca Ulker Poschl
Bahcesehir University, Institute of
Health Sciences, Physiotherapy and
Rehabilitation

Ahmet Üşen
Health Sciences University Şişli
Hamidiye Etfal Research and
Education Hospital, Istanbul, Turkey

Bilal Uysal
Bolu Physical Medicine And
Rehabilitation Hospital, Physical
Medicine And Rehabilitation
Department, Bolu, Turkey

Hayat Yalın
İstanbul Bahçeşehir University,
Faculty of Health Sciences, Nursing
Department, Istanbul, Turkey

Ilknur Yayla
Department of Nursing Management,
Acıbadem Health Group,
Istanbul, Turkey

Çiçek Duman and Feryal Subaşı

Effects of Pinch, Grip and Upper Extremity Muscle Strength on Fine Motor Skills

Abstract: *Introduction* Hand use capacity is influenced by many things such as age, gender, and coordination. Beside the importance of the understanding of these parameters' effects on hand use capacity, other demographics with possible influence on hand function need to be addressed. The aim of this study is to find out how upper extremity muscle strength and grip and pinch strength influence these parameters.

Material and Method This study included 40 voluntary students (50 % of male, 50 % of female). Upper extremity muscle strength was evaluated by Jtech Commander Power Track 2 Muscle Testing Dynamometer. Jtech Hand Grip Dynamometer and Jtech Pinch Grip Dynamometer were used for the assessment of hand grip power and finger pinch grip power, respectively. Moreover, fine motor movements were assessed by Purdue Pegboard Battery.

Results A statistically significant gender difference related to grip & pinch strength and fine motor movement scores (p<0,05) was observed. Furthermore, it is founded that all parameters of the upper extremity such as grip strength, pinch strength and fine motor skills were related to each other. While grip strength and pinch strength had a positive correlation between themselves (p<0,05), they correlated negatively with fine motor movement (p> 0,05).

Conclusion & Discussion It is founded that all parameters of the upper extremity such as grip strength, pinch strength and fine motor skills were related to each other. While grip strength and pinch strength had a positive correlation, they correlated negatively with fine motor movement. We hope that this study will assist the physiotherapists who work related to hand and upper extremity and the future studies.

Keywords: Fine Motor Skills, Grip Strength, Muscle Strength, Pinch Strength

Introduction

Human hand is one of the most complex organs that is used for grasping and carrying things to explore or manipulate. Fine motor skills are essential for these activities (1, 2). They are defined as the actions requiring degrees of control and accuracy and are controlled by the smaller muscle (3).

Hand use capacity is influenced by many things such as age, gender, and coordination (4). For example, it is a well-known fact that males and females employ different movement strategies in manual tasks, males emphasize speed of performance, whereas females emphasize accuracy (5). In another study done by

Tab. 1: Physical Characteristics of the Study Group (N = 40)

Descriptive Statistics				
	Minimum	Maximum	Mean	Standard Deviation
Age	20	25	22,83	1,152
Height (cm)	155	192	173,55	9,567
Weight (kg)	47	110	67,42	14,266
BMI	17,01	29,84	22,20	2,99872
	Right	Left		
Dominant Side	38	2		

Rodríguez-Aranda et al. (6) in 2016, movement times and kinematics were evaluated to compare hand function between different age groups and it was found that movements of older adults are both slower and qualitatively different from those of younger adults.

Beside the importance of the understanding of these parameters' effects on hand use capacity, other demographics with possible influence on hand function need to be addressed.

For example, literature says that pinch strength can be used to more accurately examine fine motor skills and task-specific grasping functions (7). However, the majority of the studies were done with children. Similarly, handgrip strength, a measure of maximum voluntary force of the hand, has been described as the simplest, valid, and reliable method in assessing muscle function, but there is a lack of study that shows the relationship between handgrip strength and hand use capacity (8).

The aim of this study is to find out how upper extremity muscle strength and grip and pinch strength influence on these parameters.

Material and Method

This study included 40 voluntary students (50 % of male, 50 % of female) studying in Yeditepe University between the period of February 2015–March 2015.

Inclusion criteria were being voluntary and being between 18 and 27 years old. Individuals who had a nerve damage or fracture in the upper extremity, who had undergone surgery on the elbow area, and who had a cognitive problem that could lead to failure to complete the tests were excluded from the study.

The mean age, height, weight, body mass index, and dominant side of individuals were given in Tab. 1.

The data was collected from self report, paper based, cross-sectional questionnaire, and clinical examination. The questionnaire focused on demographic items such as age, gender, body weight, height, dominant side, tobacco smoking, alcohol consumption, chronic diseases, use of any drug, and past surgeries.

Strength Assestments of Upper Extremity with Myometer

In clinics, manual muscle testing is generally used to measure the muscle strength because it does not require any equipment and can be done in many conditions. However, such measurement is not an objective measurement and can be affected by the muscle strength and the experience of the examiner (9).

In our study, Jtech Commander Power Track 2 Muscle Testing Dynamometer, which quantifies muscle power, was used to assess the strength of shoulder flexion, extension, abduction, adduction, internal and external rotation; elbow flexion, extension; pronation, supination; and wrist flexion, extension, ulnar and radial deviation. Test positions were similar to the goniometric measurement positions. Each measurement was repeated 3 times and the mean value was noted as the score.

Similarly, to make an objective measurement, Jtech Hand Grip Dynamometer and Jtech Pinch Grip Dynamometer were used for the assessment of hand grip power and finger pinch grip power, respectively. The volunteers were positioned in a chair with slight shoulder adduction, 90 degree elbow flexion and neutral forearm position. After the practice, they were asked to perform the grip and then pinch with all their best effort. All measurements were done for three times then the mean values were recorded to evaluate hand grip and pinch grip strength.

Fine Motor Skill Assessment

Fine motor skills are smaller movements done by the smaller muscles and usually requires control and accuracy (3,10). In our study, the standardized Purdue Pegboard Battery (model 32020, Lafayette instrument, US) was used to assess fine motor skills. It was administered according to the instructions in the test manual (11).

The Battery has two rows of 30 holes. Participants were asked to take pegs from a bowl at the top of the pegboard and to place as many pegs as in the row of holes indicated by the tester in 30 sec; first with their dominant hand, then with their nondominant hand and finally with both hands together. The score reported was the number of pegs placed for each respective condition.

In the assembly subtask, participants were asked to put together an assembly of a peg, a collar and two washers, working with both hands together. In this subtask, participants were given one minute to complete as many "assemblies" as possible. The score reported was the number of parts assembled.

A sum-score of the four pegboard subtasks was calculated to obtain a composite measure of fine motor skill.

Statistics

'Statistical Package Analyze for Social Sciences' (SPSS) version 22.0 was used for data analyses in our study. The variables were investigated using probability plots and Shapiro Wilk test to determine the normality of the distribution and were found normal (p>0,05). Descriptive statistics, mean ± standard deviation (X ± SD) were gathered. The level of significance were accepted as p≤0,05. Independent sample t-test was used to find out the relationship between gender and hand muscle strength and fine motor movements. Correlation test was used to identify the relation between upper extremity muscle strength, hand muscle strength, and fine motor movement skills.

Results

Independent sample t-test was used. Data expressed as mean ± standard deviation. Significance was set as p≤0,05.

According to the Tab. 2, there is a statistically significant difference between the male and female grip and pinch strength and fine motor movement scores except both hand Purdue Pegboard score (p<0,05).

Tab. 3 shows the correlation between fine motor movements and hand strength parameters, and BMI.

There was a negative (−) correlation between grip strength of both extremities and all Purdue Pegboard measurements (p<0,05) except the "both hands" measurements (p>0,05). At the same time, there was a negative correlation between right hand's pinch strength and Purdue Pegboard measurements, while left hand does not any kind of correlation.

Furthermore, there was a strong positive (+) correlation between BMI and grip strength of right hand and pinch strength of both extremities (p<0,01); but, there was a negative (−) correlation between BMI and Purdue Pegboard measurements (p<0,05).

When reading Tab. 4, we can see that all right-hand Purdue Pegboard scores are negatively correlated with shoulder flexor and external rotator muscle's strength while positively correlated with internal rotator, adductor and abductor muscle strength (p<0,05). Left hand Purdue Pegboard scores are positively correlated with only internal rotation muscle strength. On the other hand, any of the "both hand" measurements of Purdue Pegboard Test cannot be associated with the muscle strength.

Tab. 2: Comparison of Grip Strength, Pinch Strength and Purdue Pegboard Measurements According to the Gender (N=40)

		Women	Men		
		Mean±SD	Mean±SD	t	*p*
Grip Strength (lbs)					
	Right Hand	47,41±11,72	88,73±14,72	-9,92	**0,00***
	Left Hand	45,26±9,17	82,14±16,62	-8,68	**0,00***
Pinch Strength (lbs)					
	Right Hand	13,86±3,20	20,18±3,49	-5,95	**0,00***
	Left Hand	15,13±7,09	19,74±3,50	-2,60	**0,01***
Purdue Pegboard (pcs)					
	Right Hand	18,31±1,17	15,99±1,26	5,98	**0,00***
	Left Hand	16,43±1,24	15,14±1,41	3,04	**0,00***
	Both Hands	14,27±1,33	13,33±3,41	1,15	**0,25**
	Assembly	42,01±5,17	37,49±4,79	2,86	**0,00***

Independent Sample T-Test was used.
* Correlation is significant at the 0,05 level (two tailed).
** Correlation is significant at the 0,01 level (two tailed).
t: Independent T Test coefficient

According to the correlation test run to determine the association between Purdue Pegboard Test and distal muscle strength of upper extremity, it has been found that there is no statistically significant correlation between the "both hand" measurement and muscle strength. However, there is a negative significant correlation between the other measurements of Purdue Pegboard Test and muscle strength (p<0,05).

Discussion and Conclusion

In our study we found that BMI has a positive relationship with both grip and pinch strength (p< 0,05), while it has a negative relationship with the Purdue Pegboard measurements (p<0,05). There are so many studies supporting our results. For example, Apovian et al. (12) stated that greater hand grip strength is related to the higher BMI. Similarly, Nikolaidis et al. (13) reported that bilateral grip strength were positively associated with BMI in sports population. Additionally, D'Hondt et al. (14) stated that obese participants' fine motor skill performance was worse compared to both other BMI-groups.

Tab. 3: Correlation between Purdue Pegboard Scores and BMI, Pinch and Grip Strength (N=40)

		Pinch Strength (lbs)		Grip Strength (lbs)		BMI
		Right Hand	**Left Hand**	**Right Hand**	**Left Hand**	
Purdue Pegboard (pcs)						
Right Hand						
	r	-0,58**	-0,23	-0,59**	-0,63**	-0,53**
	p	0,00	0,13	0,00	0,00	0,00
Left Hand						
	r	-0,31*	0,13	-0,40**	-0,39*	-0,40*
	p	0,04	0,40	0,01	0,01	0,01
Both Hands						
	r	0,09	0,17	-0,00	-0,03	-0,14
	p	0,55	0,28	0,97	0,81	0,37
Assembly						
	r	-0,32*	-0,17	-0,32*	-0,37*	-0,38*
	p	0,04	0,28	0,04	0,01	0,01
BMI						
	r	0,46**	0,16	0,44**	0,53**	
	p	0,00	0,32	0,00	0,00	

Pearson correlation test was used. BMI: Body Mass Index.
* Correlation is significant at the 0,05 level (two tailed).
** Correlation is significant at the 0,01 level (two tailed).
r: Pearson's correlation coefficient

Literature says that fine motor performance of children depends on many factors such as hand muscle strength, grip and pinch strength, muscle tone, joint range of motion, and coordination (15). This data was different to the achieved data for adults in this study, which found that when pinch or grasp strength increases (except left hand pinch strength), Purdue Pegboard scores (except both hands) decrease (p = 0,05). Also, there are some other studies claiming that gross grasp strength did not appear to have a significant contribution to fine motor control (16). It could be considered as the literature mostly focused on people with some kind of diseases such as cognitive, rheumatic, or diseases with spasticity, but our study was conducted with healthy people. Furthermore, muscles that control fine movements and require precise but low strength have fewer fibers per motor unit, while the large muscles that control gross motor movements requiring greater strength may contain greater numbers of muscle

Tab. 4: Correlation between Purdue Pegboard Scores and Shoulder Muscle Strength (N=40)

			Right Hand	Left Hand	Both Hands	Assembly
			Purdue Pegboard (pcs)			
Flexion						
S	R	r	-0,69**	-0,45**	-0,12	-0,50**
H		p	0,00	0,00	0,44	0,00
O	L	r	-0,64**	-0,40*	-0,15	-0,50**
U		p	0,00	0,01	0,34	0,00
L **Extension**						
D	R	r	-0,48**	0,25	-0,20	-0,36*
E		p	0,00	0,11	0,19	0,01
R	L	r	0,54**	-0,26	-0,17	-0,31*
		p	0,00	0,10	0,28	0,04
Abduction						
	R	r	0,59**	-0,35*	-0,11	-0,45**
		p	0,00	0,02	0,48	0,00
	L	r	0,54**	-0,32*	-0,09	-0,41**
		p	0,00	0,04	0,56	0,00
Adduction						
	R	r	0,42**	-0,25	0,00	-0,34*
		p	0,00	0,12	0,96	0,03
	L	r	0,37*	-0,21	0,02	-0,40*
		p	0,01	0,19	0,87	0,01
Internal Rotation						
	R	r	0,51**	-0,44**	-0,12	-0,36*
		p	0,00	0,00	0,46	0,02
	L	r	0,63**	0,47**	-0,26	-0,45**
		p	0,00	0,00	0,09	0,00
External Rotation						
	R	r	-0,56**	-0,46**	-0,03	-0,46**
		p	0,00	0,00	0,84	0,00
	L	r	-0,53**	-0,41**	-0,28	-0,41**
		p	0,00	0,00	0,07	0,00

Pearson correlation test was used. R: Right, L: Left.
* Correlation is significant at the 0,05 level (two tailed).
** Correlation is significant at the 0,01 level (two tailed).
r: Pearson's correlation coefficient

Tab. 5: Correlation between Purdue Pegboard Scores and Elbow, Forearm and Wrist Muscle Strength (N=40)

				Purdue Pegboard (pcs)			
				Right Hand	Left Hand	Both Hands	Assembly
	Flexion						
E		R	r	-0,60**	-0,28	-0,26	-0,50**
L			p	0,00	0,07	0,10	0,00
B		L	r	-0,57**	-0,33*	-0,09	-0,48**
O			p	0,00	0,03	0,56	0,00
W	**Extension**						
		R	r	-0,61**	-0,44**	-0,24	-0,46**
			p	0,00	0,00	0,12	0,00
		L	r	-0,55**	-0,44**	-0,24	-0,41**
			p	0,00	0,00	0,13	0,00
	Pronation						
F		R	r	-0,50**	-0,30*	-0,01	-0,35*
O			p	0,00	0,05	0,93	0,02
R		L	r	-0,37*	-0,23	0,01	-0,31*
E			p	0,01	0,14	0,91	0,04
A	**Supination**						
R		R	r	-0,52**	-0,33*	0,00	-0,41**
M			p	0,00	0,03	0,99	0,00
		L	r	-0,37*	-0,39*	0,12	-0,36*
			p	0,01	0,01	0,42	0,02
	Flexion						
W		R	r	-0,56**	-0,33*	-0,04	-0,47**
R			p	0,00	0,03	0,78	0,000
I							
S							
T		L	r	-0,52**	-0,31*	-0,12	-0,56**
			p	0,00	0,05	0,45	0,00
	Extension						
		R	r	-0,49**	-0,26	-0,11	-0,50**
			p	0,00	0,10	0,48	0,00
		L	r	-0,56**	-0,30*	-0,12	-0,57**
			p	0,00	0,05	0,43	0,00
	Ulnar Deviation						
		R	r	-0,50**	-0,26	-0,15	-0,30
			p	0,00	0,09	0,32	0,06
		L	r	-0,58**	-0,48**	-0,10	-0,54**
			p	0,00	0,00	0,51	0,00

Tab. 5: (continued)

			Purdue Pegboard (pcs)			
Radial Deviation						
	R	r	-0,46**	-0,33*	-0,18	-0,33*
		p	0,00	0,03	0,91	0,03
	L	r	-0,47**	-0,26	-0,03	-0,36*
		p	0,00	0,09	0,84	0,02

Pearson correlation test was used. R: Right, L: Left.
* Correlation is significant at the 0,05 level (two tailed).
** Correlation is significant at the 0,01 level (two tailed).
r: Pearson's correlation coefficient

fibers (17). This may be another reason why the hand muscle strength is negatively related with the fine motor skills.

There are so many studies that claim that fine motor skills require stronger upper extremity muscles. In a study done by Kılınç et al. (18) in 2013, 60 subjects with muscle weakness were evaluated by many different evaluation methods including dynamometric muscle strength, grip strength, and Minnesota hand dexterity test (MHDT). They found a significant correlation between upper extremity muscle strength and functional evaluation methods. Similarly, in our study, the positive correlation between the fine motor ability and right shoulder abduction, adduction and internal rotation strength can be explained by this theory.

We also examined the hand muscle strength and fine motor skill differences between two genders. Our study supports the literature and proved there is a statistically significant difference between two genders related to hand muscle strength and fine motor movements. In the literature, there are many studies related to gender differences. For example, in a study done by Ruff et al. (19) in 1993, 360 healthy volunteers divided into groups according to their age and gender and their eye-hand coordination and motor speed were investigated. They revealed that the finger-tapping test evaluating muscle motor speed showed significant gender differences, since women were substantially slower and in the Grooved Pegboard Test, evaluating fine motor movements, women were found substantially faster than men. In our study, only the "both hand" score was not significant and this might be due to the difficulty of bilateral coordination tasks for both genders. However, following studies are needed to prove how bilateral movements changes for both genders.

As a conclusion, it is founded that all parameters of the upper extremity such as grip strength, pinch strength and fine motor skills were related to each other.

While grip strength and pinch strength had a positive correlation, they correlated negatively with fine motor movement.

Limitations

Although the lower sample size is the limitation of our study, we hope that this study will assist the physiotherapists who work related to hand and upper extremity and the future studies.

Conflict of Interest

The authors declare no conflict of interest by the authors.

Disclosure Statement

We would like to state that the above-mentioned manuscript has not been published elsewhere, has not been accepted for publication elsewhere, or under editorial review for publication elsewhere.

Financial Disclosure

The authors declared that they did not receive financial support for this study.

References

1. Kim, B. J., Bishu, R. R. (2004) Grasp at Submaximal Strength. In: Kumar, S. *Muscle Strength* (pp 213–226). USA: CRC Press LLC.
2. Allgöwer K, Hermsdörfer J. (2017) Fine Motor Skills Predict Performance in the Jebsen Taylor Hand Function Test after Stroke. *Clin Neurophysiol.* 128(10): 1858–1871. doi: 10.1016/j.clinph.2017.07.408.
3. Donald, D. E., Pinson, J. (2012) *Music Therapy in Principle and Practice* (2nd Ed.), USA: Charles C Thomas Publisher.
4. Fagarasanu, M., Kumar, S. (2004) Hand Strength. In: Kumar, S. *Muscle Strength*, USA: CRC Press LLC.
5. Rohr, L. E. (2006). Gender-Specific Movement Strategies Using a Computerpointing Task. *Journal of Motor Behavior*, 38(6), 431–437.
6. Rodríguez-Aranda, C., Mittner, M., & Vasylenko, O. (2016). Association between Executive Functions, Working Memory, and Manual Dexterity in Young and Healthy Older Adults: An Exploratory Study. *Perceptual and Motor Skills*, 122(1), 165–192.

7. Shultz, S. J., Houglum, P. A., Perrin, D. H. (2016) *Examination of Musculoskeletal Injuries with Web Resource* (4th Ed.). USA: Human Kinetics.
8. Cuesta-Vargas, A., Hilgenkamp, T. (2015) Reference Values of Grip Strength Measured with a Jamar Dynamometer in 1526 Adults with Intellectual Disabilities and Compared to Adults without Intellectual Disability. *PLoS ONE*, 10(6). doi:10.1371/journal.pone.0129585.
9. Clarkson Hazel, M. (2000) *Musculoskeletal Assessment: Joint Range of Motion and Manual Muscle Strength* (2nd Ed.). USA: Lippincott Williams & Wilkins.
10. Pickup, I., Price, L. (2007) *Teaching Physical Education in the Primary School: A Developmental Approach.* Great Britain: Bell & Bain Ltd.
11. Lafayette Instrument (2002) Purdue Pegboard Test – Model 32020 User Instructions. 1–42.
12. Apovian, C. M., Frey, C. M., Wood, G. C. et al. (2002) Mass Index and Physical Function in Older Women. *Obesity Research*, 10(8), 740-747.
13. Nikolaïdis, P. (2012) Development of Isometric Muscular Strength in Adolescent Soccer Players. *Physical Education and Sport*, 10(3), 231–242.
14. D'Hondt, E., Deforche, B., De Bourdeaudhuij, I., Lenoir, M. (2008) Childhood Obesity Affects Fine Motor Skill Performance under Different Postural Constraints. *Neuroscience Letters*, 440(1), 72–77. doi:10.1016/j. neulet.2008.05.056
15. Mulligan, S. E. (2014) *Occupational Therapy Evaluation for Children: A Pocket Guide* (2nd Ed.). China: Lippincott Williams & Wilkins.
16. Squillace, M., Ray, S., Milazzo, M. (2015) Changes in Gross Grasp Strength and Fine Motor Skills in Adolescents with Pediatric Multiple Sclerosis. *Occup Ther Health Care*, 29 (1): 77–85. doi: 10.3109/07380577.2014.967441.
17. Kuriki, H. U., De Azevedo, F. M., Takahashi, L. S. O. et al. (2012). The Relationship between Electromyography and Muscle Force. In: Schwartz, M. (eds.) *EMG Methods for Evaluating Muscle and Nerve Function* (pp. 31–54). China: InTech.
18. Kılınç, M., Aksu Yıldırım, S. A., Kayıhan, H. (2013) Erişkin Nöromusküler Hastalıklarda Üst Ekstremite Fonksiyonlarını Değerlendiren Yöntemlerin Karşılaştırılması. *Ergoterapi ve Rehabilitasyon Dergisi*, 1 (1): 1–8.
19. Ruff, R. M., & Parker, S. B. (1993). Gender- and Age-Specific Changes in Motor Speed and Eye-Hand Coordination in Adults: Normative Values for the Finger Tapping and Grooved Pegboard Tests. *Perceptual and Motor Skills*, 76(3_suppl), 1219–1230. doi:10.2466/pms.1993.76.3c.1219

Gonca Ulker Poschl, Dilber Karagozoglu Coskunsu,
and H. Serap Inal

Investigation of the Relationship between Physical Activity Level and Postural Changes in Adolescents

Abstract: This study aims to evaluate postural disorders and physical activity levels of adolescents between 14 and 17 years of age. This study included 100 voluntary students (mean age 16.0±0.7 years) attending St. George Austrian High School. Students' physical activity levels were assessed with International Physical Activity Questionnaire-Short Form (IPAQ-SF); postures were evaluated with New York Posture Rating Test (NYPRT) and symmetrigraph; pain levels were assessed with Cornell Musculoskeletal Discomfort Questionnaire. According to our results, regular physical exercise habit was present in 67.3 % of males and 78.4 % of females. Based on IPAQ criteria, 10 % of the participants were inactive, 54 % were minimally active, and 36 % were highly active. Students' postures were evaluated according to NYPRT criteria, and the most frequent postural disorders among females were anterior tilt of the head (44.9 %), increased lumbar lordosis (40.8 %), uneven shoulder levels (32.7 %), and shoulder protraction (32.7 %); whereas anterior tilt of the head (67.4 %), shoulder protraction (51.0 %) and thoracic kyphosis (48.9 %) were most frequently observed among males. One of the most common postural disorders among females and males was pes planus. The most frequent areas causing pain were back (32.9 %), lower back (22.4 %) and neck (14.3 %) among females, and back (31.4 %), lower back (14.7 %) and right shoulder (11.8 %) among males. We found that the majority of students had high physical activity levels, which we believe may be related to having conducted the study in a private school. In adolescents, it is important to acquire a habit of doing regular physical exercise in order to maintain the favorable effects of physical activity on posture. Prolonged sitting adversely affects the posture.

Keywords: Adolescent, Physical activity, Sport, Posture New York Posture, Symmetrigraph

Introduction

Posture, as the combinations of static and dynamic positions defines the relationship of body parts with each other and with the entire body (1) and is considered as good or normal if the balance between musculoskeletal system structures is optimum and, the body structures are under the least pressure during motion and in resting (2). In other words, good posture is one of the signs of a healthy musculoskeletal system. The muscular imbalances or postural changes may increase the forces falling on the body parts and may lead to different postural disorders at different levels in course of time (3). Adolescence stage, which is regarded as the passage from childhood to adulthood (13–17 years) is also encountered as the period when postural disorders frequently start because it is the period when biological, cognitive, and physical changes most rapidly appear (4). The sedentary life style and the absence of regular physical activity (PA) habits are the main issues that accelerate these postural problems (5,6). Additionally, insufficient PA leads to postural disorders that may be associated with different chronic health problems, and increases the risks for the life-threatening chronic diseases as diabetes, hypertension, cardiovascular diseases, obesity, and cancer (7,8,9). Therefore, it has been reported that acquiring the habit of regular PA as much as possible in early ages, as well as maintaining this during adolescence ages are the most important requirements for the physical and mental health of the individuals (7,10,11). Accordingly, a daily PA performed at least 60 min (7 days a week) regularly is recommended for children between 6 and 17 years of age and for adolescents (10,11). However, it is reported that despite the physically active childhood, especially girls tend to have a decrease in their PA level towards the adolescence ages (12,13). This may be in relation to the time limitations due to assignments and preparations to high school/university entrance examinations in Turkey. Since in most large cities in Turkey, students are using transportation provided by their parents or the school administration, their daily walking duration is also limited. The need to spare extra time among their academic duties as well as the cost for participating in sports activities may be the other common barriers for joining the regular PA programs. Thus, the physical education (PE) classes may be the only PA that the adolescents may practice weekly. Unfortunately, the recent national literature supports these ideas, reporting that among the 319 adolescent students 79 % were physically inactive (14), and only 49.7 % of adolescents were regularly engaged in sports activities but their mean weekly time spent was limited to only 2.05 hours (15). Additionally, it was reported that among the high school students only 45.8 % were physically inactive and they were having musculoskeletal pain complaints (16). The authors stated that the main complaint were neck and back pain among inactive students, especially among girls. However, it was not mentioned whether the pain felt was associated with their postural problems or not, additionally, if there was relationship between physical activity level and the posture of the adolescents. Therefore, we aimed to evaluate the relationship between physical activity level and postural disorders in adolescence (14–17 years).

Material and Method

The ninth and tenth grade students (n = 101) attending to a high school in the academic year 2016–2017 participated in the study between February 2017 and March 2017. All that were studying in the high school were suitable to the inclusion criteria, being between the age of 14 and 17 years and accepting to participate in the study. The presence of a disorder that would affect the posture of a student and having a history of surgery or trauma were the exclusion criteria. One student was excluded from the study due to prior hip surgery and related unequal leg length. The rest were informed about the aim and the procedures of the study, informed consent forms were read and signed by the families of the participants.

All the participants were evaluated by the physiotherapist-PT (GUP) in a specially designed assessment room under the knowledge of their teacher in the school environment.

Assessments

Sociodemographic and Physical Activity Habit

A specially designed form to assess their sociodemographic features (weight-kg and height-cm, and body mass index-BMI-kg/m^2), their habit of regular sports activities as hourly, daily and/or weekly, the type of school as bag backpack, shoulder bag, handbag and other, and the habit of carrying their bags as on one shoulder, in one hand, hung on both shoulders posteriorly, and others was used to gather the information.

According to their class schedules, the time spent sitting at school were determined. The total time spent out of the school, that is, sitting outside the school and home and at the desk (homework, internet use, computer homework) or in the couch (television, books, iPad) were searched and recorded to the same form.

Assessment of Posture

New York Posture Rating (NYPR) test and symmetrigraph were used for evaluating the posture of the students. In addition, Adams test was used for investigating scoliosis.

NYPR test, which was originally developed for the assessment of postural status of the children attending schools in New York State, was used to evaluate the alignment disorders that can be seen in 13 regions in the body. The best suitable one of three different images in the test form was selected by the PT for each body region, and was scored as "5" for normal alignment, "3" for mild deviation, and "1" for marked deviation (17).

Total maximum score that could be obtained at the end of the assessment was 65 and the minimum score was 13. Standard evaluation value was "very good" if total score was greater than or equal to 45, "good" if it was between 40 and 44, "fair" if it was between 30 and 39, "poor" if it was between 20 and 29, and "bad" if it was less than 19 (18).

It has been reported that NYPR is a practical assessment method with moderate intra-class correlation coefficient (0.70) but low inter-rater correlation coefficient (0.57), and it is more reliable if it is used by the same rater for repeated assessments (19).

In order to increase the sensitivity of the assessment in our study, a transparent posture chart 2 meters long and 1 meter wide and divided into 6-cm squares was used for posture analysis (symmetrigraph). The body was evaluated from the posterior to lateral with the aid of a red line drawn perpendicular to the floor on the symmetrigraph (18) (Fig. 1).

Thus, a more sensitive assessment could be made by means of the red reference line and squares. For equal assessment of all individuals, the symmetrigraph was fixated to the floor of the assessment room. Each student was evaluated by standing on the marked point 1.5 m away from the symmetrigraph. For posterior posture analysis, the student was positioned as for the reference line (RL) to pass from the mid-points of both shoulders and heels and above the spine,and for lateral analysis, the RL passing 2 cm in front of the lateral malleolus. Before the assessment, the students were asked to take off their clothes above their waist, and the females to wear a tight t-shirt, remove their shoes, look straight ahead, and stand in a position where they felt comfortable. First, posterior analysis was carried out. Then the students were asked to turn 90° over the marked point to have the symmetrigraph on their left side and lateral analysis was carried out.

In addition, Adams test, which is a rapid and efficient method used in schools for screening lateral deviations of spine if it is functional or structural to support the outcomes of the NYPR test, was used. While the physiotherapist (GUP) stood behind the student, the student was asked to bend forward with knees in extension and both hands joined and the back parallel to the floor. The spine was analyzed horizontally to see whether there was a rip hump on the deformed side of the back indicating gibbosity or not, and if there was no rip hump on the back of the student, this meant even if the student had a lateral deviation of the spine according to the NYPR test, this was not structural (20).

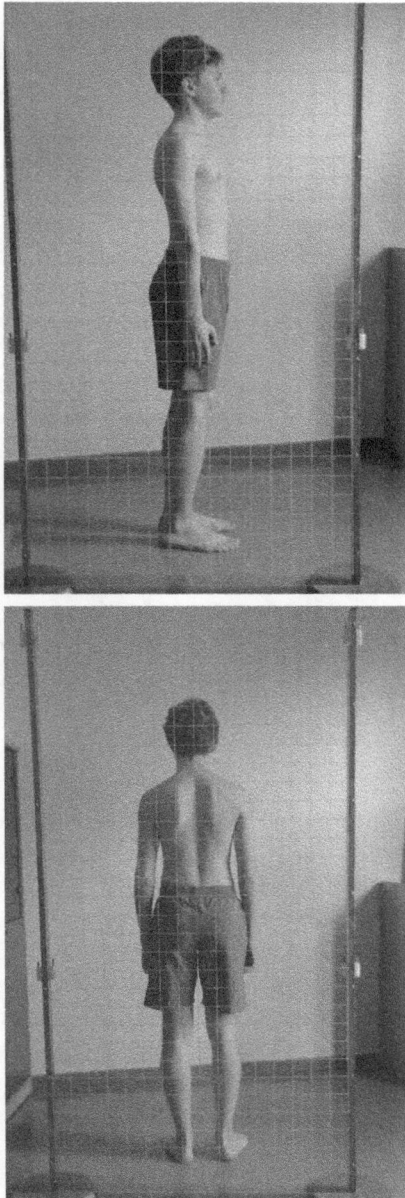

Fig. 1: Posture Analysis: a) Lateral b) Posterior. Written consent was obtained from the guardian of the student for taking his photograph and using it.

Cornell Musculoskeletal Discomfort Questionnaire

Musculoskeletal pain was assessed by subtype of the Turkish version of Cornell musculoskeletal discomfort questionnaire, which was adapted for students to observe their pain or discomfort in 11 separate body regions (instead of 20 as it was in the original) during the last seven days as well as to understand the frequency and severity of their pain (21, 22).

The students were assessed by face-to-face questions and were asked to select the suitable answer to express the frequency of their pain as "none felt, 1–2 times during the week, 3–4 times during the week, once every day, many times every day," to determine the severity of pain as "mild, moderate, very severe"; and to determine whether it hindered their studying or not by selecting one of the followings as "did not hinder, hindered a little, hindered a lot".

When the frequency of feeling pain was scored, the answers of "none felt, 1–2 times during the week, 3–4 times during the week, once every day, many times every day" were scored "0, 1.5, 3.5, 5, 10" points, respectively.

When the severity of pain was scored, "1, 2, 3" points were given to the answers of "mild, moderate, very severe", respectively.

Hindrance of studying for lessons was scored "1, 2, 3" points for the answers of "did not hinder, hindered a little, hindered a lot", respectively. Total score of frequency of feeling pain, severity of pain, and hindrance of studying for lessons forms the Cornell Musculoskeletal Discomfort Questionnaire score (21).

International Physical Activity Questionnaire – Short Form (IPAQ-SF)

The Turkish version consisting of 7 questions (23) in the International Physical Activity Questionnaire (IPAQ) (24), which provides information about walking, moderate, severe physical activity, and sitting time, was used in the study.

For calculating the short form, durations, frequencies, and metabolic equivalent (MET) values of sitting, walking, moderate activities (carrying light objects, cycling at normal pace, folk dancing, dancing, bowling, playing tennis) and severe activities (lifting heavy objects, digging, doing aerobics, playing basketball, playing football, cycling fast) were multiplied and weekly MET-minute/week scores of the individuals were obtained.

Standard MET values for these physical activities are given below:

Walking = 3.3 MET,
Moderate Physical Activity = 4.0 MET,
Severe Physical Activity = 8.0 MET,

Total MET-minute/week scores of the individuals are obtained by using these values and with the sum of walking, sitting, moderate and severe activity scores. According to the score of this questionnaire, physical activity levels of individuals are evaluated in 3 categories as "inactive", "minimally active" and "very active".

Physically inactive <600 MET-minute / week
Low physical activity level 600–3000 MET-minute / week
High physical activity level 3000 MET-minute / week and above (24).

Statistical Analysis

"Statistical Package for Social Sciences" (SPSS) Version 20 (SPSS Inc, Chicago, IL, USA) statistical program and Microsoft Excel 2016 were used for analyzing study data. Statistical significance level was evaluated at the level of p<0.05 for all statistical analyses. Normality of the distribution of data groups was determined with the "Kolmogorow–Smirnow" test in order to select suitable advanced statistical analyses for analyzing study data. Non-parametric "Mann–Whitney-U" test was used because distribution of data groups was not normal. "Spearman Correlation" test was used for correlation analysis.

Consent and Ethics

After obtaining consent from TR Beyoğlu County National Education Directorate for carrying out the assessment, ethics consent was obtained from the Ethics Committee of Bahçeşehir University (dating March 01, 2017 and 2017–04/03 number). The study was conducted in accordance with Helsinki Declaration regulations.

Results

All the students spent the same time sitting in the class while listening to their lessons, which was 6 hours.

In order to investigate the relationship between physical activity and posture in adolescents, 101 ninth and tenth grade students aged between 14 and 17 years were invited to the study. Assessments were made in February–March 2017. One student was excluded from the study due to prior hip surgery and related unequal leg length. Demographic and physical characteristics of 100 students included in the study are shown in Tab. 1.

Right hand was the dominant hand in 87.8 % of girls (n=43) and in 88.2 % of boys (n=45).

Tab. 1: Demographic and Physical Properties of Individuals

	Females (n=49)			Males (n=51)		p
	(mean±std)			(mean±std)		
Age *(years)*	16,0±0,6			15,9±0,7		0,29
Body mass index *(kg/m²)*	21,1±2,2			22,2±3,0		0,03
Grouping according to body mass index	**Thin**	**Normal**	**Fat**	**Thin**	**Normal**	**Fat**
Number (n), percentage (%)	0	44	5	1	35	15
	(0 %)	(89,8 %)	(10,2 %)	(2 %)	(68,6 %)	(28,4 %)
Mann Whitney U						

Tab. 2: Rates and Durations of Sports Activities

	Female	Male	p
Doing sports regularly (percentage)	67,3 %	78,4 %	0,21
Duration of sports activity (hours)	3,91	5,54	0,03
Duration of regular sports habit (years)	3,66	3,39	0,31
Mann Whitney U			

All the students carried bags on their way to school, 97.96 % of girls and 98.04 % of boys had backpacks and the rest used shoulder bags. **Sports Habits:** Rates and durations of sports activities are shown in **Tab. 2**.

Distribution of types of sports performed by the students is shown in **Fig. 2**. The students were engaged in 20 different types of sports activities. Girls were engaged mostly in fitness, volleyball, dancing, and pilates, while boys in fitness, basketball, and swimming.

Weekly sports activities of students doing sports regularly are shown in Fig. 3.

Most of the students performed sports for a range of 2–3 hours weekly.

Duration of doing sports in years is shown in Fig. 4. Females who were engaged in sports for more than 9 years performed ballet or swimming starting from a very young age and males acquired the habit of doing sports for 10 years or more with swimming. Another fact identified during assessments is that postures and muscular elasticity of the students who were engaged in ballet or swimming were better than the others.

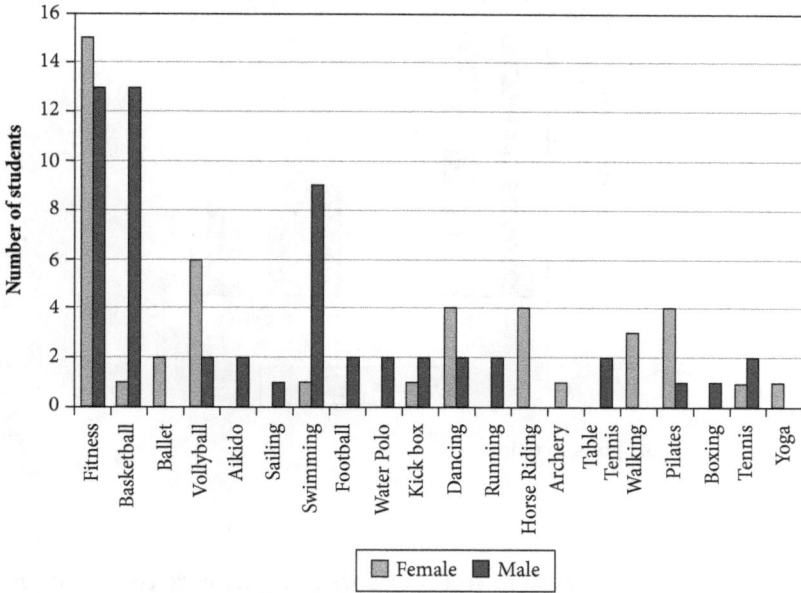

Fig. 2: Distribution of Types of Sports

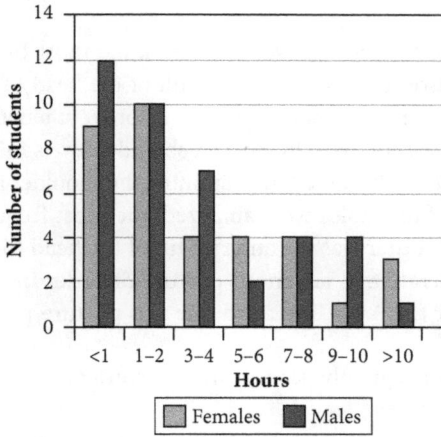

Fig. 3: Weekly Sports Activities

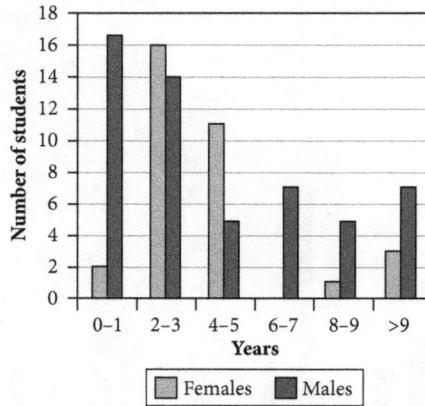

Fig. 4: Duration of Sports Activities

Posture

When total New York posture scores of boys and girls were compared, there was a significant difference in favor of the females (p=0,010) where the posture of all females (n=49) was very good while the posture scores of males were as follows: 92,2 % (n=47) was very good, 5,9 % (n=3) was good, and 2 % (n=1) was poor.

When postures of the females were analyzed, the most frequent moderate or advanced posture disorder was the anterior tilt of the head (44.9 %). The second most frequent moderate and advanced posture disorder in females was noted in the back (40.8 %). This was followed by uneven shoulder levels (32.7 %) and protraction of the shoulder (32.7 %) noted by examining the shoulder from the posterior.

When postures of the males were analyzed, the most frequent moderate and advanced posture disorder was the anterior tilt of the head (67.4 %). The second most frequent moderate and advanced posture disorder in males was protraction of the shoulder (51.0 %). The third one was posture problem of the upper back (48.9 %).

One of the most frequently seen posture disorders in females and males is "pes planus".

When the groups were compared regarding New York posture test regions, hip asymmetry (p=0,044), pes planus (p=0,016), anterior tilt of the head (p=0,032), chest deformity (p=0,015), thoracic kyphosis (p=0,000), protracted abdomen (p= 0,01) were significantly more common in males (Tab. 3).

Tab. 3: Comparison of New York Posture Region Scores

Mean Rank

	Female	Male	z	p
Head	51,4	49,64	-0,539	0,590
Shoulder posterior	53,86	47,27	-1,369	0,171
Spine	52,93	48,17	-1,206	0,228
Hip	53,97	47,17	-2,011	0,044
Foot	54,52	46,64	-2,410	0,016
Foot arcus	55,29	45,90	-1,840	0,066
Neck	56,11	45,11	-2,142	0,032
Chest	54,94	46,24	-2,425	0,015
Shoulder lateral	54,33	46,82	-1,507	0,132
Upper back	59,44	41,91	-3,797	0,000
Torso	52,39	48,69	-0,838	0,402
Abdomen	55,50	45,70	-3,249	0,001
Back	48,70	52,23	-0,724	0,469
Mann Whitney U				

Adams Test

There was no significant difference between the groups regarding presence of gibbosity (p=0.094). Seven males and two females had a finding of gibbosity.

Cornell Musculoskeletal Discomfort Questionnaire

There was no significant difference between the groups regarding the results of Cornell musculoskeletal discomfort questionnaire (p=0,783).

In females, pain was the most frequently seen in the back (32.9 %), lower back (22.4 %), and neck (14.3 %). In males, the areas where pain was seen most frequently were back (31.4 %), lower back (14.7 %), and right shoulder (11.8 %). The participants reported their pain to be of mild severity that did not prevent them from studying.

International Physical Activity Questionnaire

When total scores of International Physical Activity Questionnaire were compared, there was a highly significant difference between the groups (p=0,00). Males had a higher level of physical activity than females. Although 49 % (n=25) of the males were very active, 47,1 % (n=24) were minimally active and 3,9 %

(n=2) were inactive; only 22,4 % (n=11) of the female were very active, 61,2 % (n=30) were minimally active, and 16,3 % (n=8) were inactive.

Distribution of activity levels according to the scales determined by the physical activity questionnaire is shown below.

Mean sitting time of the females was 8.2 hours and that of males was 8.4 hours. When sitting times of both groups were compared, there was no significant difference (p=0,843).

Correlation of Posture Test with Other Parameters

When *Spearman* correlation coefficients regarding the relationship among variables of females was taken into consideration, there was a mildly significant positive correlation between PA levels and NYPR test variables (r=0,297; p<0,05). This was similar among males, and, also we found a mildly significant positive correlation between PA level and NYPR test variables (r=0,321; p<0,05). However, there was a mildly significant negative correlation between sitting and NYPR test variables (r=-0,354; p<0,05), and a moderately significant negative correlation between sitting and physical activity level (r=-0,427; p<0,05) only among males.

Discussion

In this study it was aimed to investigate the relationship between the level of physical activity and posture in adolescents aged 14–17. The habit of performing sports activities regularly and physical activity scores were also higher among boy students. Rate of doing regular sports was 67.3 % in girls and 78.4 % in boys and these rates are much higher than those reported in the literature that is consistent with the literature (14,15,27,28). However, the BMI of male students was higher as 10 % of girls and 29 % of boys were overweight. Tekgül et al. (2012) (25) stated that BMIs of boys performing sports regularly were within the normal limits. Thus, the other considerations such as nutrition or sitting duration may be important while searching the causes of higher BMI among adolescents. Since the study was carried out in a school that students are coming from families with a high socio-economic status may be the other issue increasing the higher rate of being overweight among adolescents (29).

It was found that students participated in 20 different sports activities ranging from ballet to kick box. When the literature is reviewed, it is seen that football (37.9 %) and basketball (18.1 %) are the most frequently practiced sports in adolescents; these sports activities are followed by walking (10 %), volleyball

(8.8 %), and handball (8.2 %) (15). Engagement in indoor sports activities mostly can be associated with the fact that they come from families with high socioeconomic income (29).

Although time spent doing regular sports and rate of physical activity was much more in boys, girls had much better posture scores in New York rating test. While posture of girls was "very good" (100 %), only 92.2 % of boys had "very good" postures and the remaining 5.9 % had "good" and 2 % had "poor" postures. Students who practiced in ballet and swimming had better postures than the other students. In the girls, the most frequent posture disorders were anterior tilt of the head (44.9 %), increased lumbar lordosis (40.8 %), uneven shoulders (32.7 %), and shoulder protraction (32.7 %). In the boys, the most frequent posture disorders were anterior tilt of the head (67.4 %), shoulder protraction (51.0 %), and thoracic kyphosis (48.9 %). Anterior tilt of the head, thoracic kyphosis, protracted abdomen and pes planus were significantly more frequent in boys compared to the girls. Pes planus was one of the most frequent posture disorders seen in both sexes. In the study by Macialczyk-Paprocka (2017) (30), investigating the prevalence of improper posture with excessive weight and obesity, shoulder protraction, increased thoracic kyphosis, genu valgum, and pes planus were more frequent in overweight and obese adolescents in the 13–18-year age group. These results are partially compatible with the results of our male students with higher BMIs. Latalski et al. (2013) (5) have reported that girls do their homework while lying in a prone position while boys prefer doing their homework at desk, which help explain the postural differences between boys and girls. Since pes planus is expected to decrease in both sexes after the ages of 5–11 (31) or 9–15 (32), we believe that the problem of flat feet found in our study needs to be emphasized because the participants in our study were above these age limits (14–17 years).

Although the level of physical activity was higher in boys, their worse postures suggest that factors other than physical activity affect the posture in a negative way. BMI was shown as a negative factor affecting posture in the literature (5,9). On the other hand, sitting position can also determine the occurrence of anterior tilt of the head which is also seen in girls though more frequently in boys and shoulder protraction and thoracic kyphosis seen in boys. In order to keep looking at a monitor below the visual field for a long time during computer, iPad, and telephone use, the head needs to be moved forward. It was suggested that this increases the anterior angulation of lower cervical vertebrae and leads to the development of anterior tilt of the head with increased posterior angulation in upper thoracal vertebrae to keep the balance (33). It has been reported that prolonged anterior tilt of the head leads to the musculoskeletal system disorder known as "upper cross syndrome" characterized with decreased lordosis in the lower cervical region, increased kyphosis in upper thoracic vertebrae, and round shoulders (34). Anterior tilt of the head can also lead to musculoskeletal system problems by affecting the thoracic spine and shoulder region (35). Although we have not searched for the presence of "upper cross syndrome", we may suggest this to be observed for the adolescents that have tendency to use technological tools (36).

The sitting time of the students were evaluated and we have not found any difference between boys and girls regarding to their sitting time. The time spent using technology and posture during sitting was not evaluated, which could be considered as the limitation of the study. Nevertheless, the presence of posture disorders even in girls with high physical activity levels and normal level of BMIs suggests that posture during sitting should also be investigated, considering the increasing dependence on technology. Although the habit of doing sports regularly and level of physical activity in girls are higher than the rates reported in the literature, the presence of posture problems like the anterior tilt of the head suggests that posture during sitting is also important in both female and male adolescents (37). In addition to the negative correlation found between the posture and sitting time, as was reported by Corder et al. (2015) (13), the decreased interest in physical activity in adolescence also has an increasing effect on sitting time.

Although no correlation was found between pain symptoms and posture scores and the pain felt was at mild level, back and lower back pain is predominant in both sexes. We assume that this may be associated with the sitting position of the students. It has been shown in the literature that the type of bag used, weight of the bag and its carrying time negatively affect posture (26). In this study, 97–98 % of the students carried backpacks. However, because they did not carry books in their bags and carried their bags for a very short time (from school to school service or private car), it was noted that bags would not affect their posture.

Conclusion

According to the results of our study, rates of doing regular sports and levels of physical activity and BMIs in adolescent boys aged between 14 and 17 years were much higher compared to the girls. Significantly higher rates of anterior tilt of the head, thoracic kyphosis, protracted abdomen, and pes planus can be associated with more than normal BMIs in boys. Although posture scores were within normal limits, we think that families and especially health education teachers should be educated and informed about common posture disorders (37) and that investigation of the time spent using technology and postures of adolescents would be helpful. On the other hand, the rates of the students playing sportsat the school where our study was conducted may not be compatible with Turkey in general. Conducting the study in many states and private schools in big cities like Istanbul and in the schools in rural areas is important for understanding the relationship between physical activity level and posture disorders in adolescence in Turkey.

Study Limitations

The limitation of our study is the small number of subjects. Our number of subjects could only be 100 because the number of students at the school where the study was conducted was small although only one student was excluded because of uneven leg height following surgery. Evaluation of more students in adolescence will enable a better understanding of the relationship between physical activity and posture.

Conflict of Interest

None.
This article has not been presented in any congress or symposium and has not been published in any other publications.

Acknowledgment

We would like to thank Werner Poschl, a teacher of St. Georg Austrian High School, for his great support and help in our study.

References

1. Blanpied, P. R. (2010). *Biomechanical Principles*. In: *Kinesiology of the Musculoskeletal System. Foundations for Rehabilitation*. London: Mosby Elsevier, 77–118.

2. Macpherson, J. M. and Horak, F. B. (2013). Posture. In: *Principles of Neuralscience*. Fifth Edition. Eric R. Kandel, James H. Schwartz, Thomas M. Jessell, Steven A. Siegelbaum, A.J. Hudspeth (Eds.). New York: McGraw Hill Medical, 935–959.

3. Lafond, D., Descarreaux, M., Normand, M. C., & Harrison, D. E. (2007). Postural Development in School Children: A Cross-Sectional Study. *Chiropractic & Osteopathy*, 15, 1. doi:10.1186/1746-1340-15-1

4. Brzęk, A., Sołtys, J., Gallert-Kopyto, W., Gwizdek, K. & Plinta R. (2016). Body Posture in Children with Obesity - the Relationship to Physical Activity (PA). *Pediatr Endocrinol Diabetes Metab*, 22(4), 148–155. doi: 10.18544/PEDM-22.04.0063

5. Latalski, M. B. J., Fatyga, M., Repko, M., Filipovic, M., Jarosz, M. J., Borowicz, K. B., Matuszewski, Ł. & Trzpis, T. (2013). Risk Factors of Postural Defects in Children at School Age. *Ann Agric Environ Med*, 3(20), 583–587.

6. Quka, N., Stratoberdha, D. H., & Selenica, R. (2015). Risk Factors of Poor Posture in Children and Its Prevalence. *Academic Journal of Interdisciplinary Studies*, 4(3), 97–102. doi: 10.5901/ajis.2015.v4n3p97

7. Organization WH. Global Recommendations on Physical Activity for Health; 2010.

8. Motow-Czyż, M., Orczyk, A. & Orczyk, M. (2014). Postural Defects Correction in the Process of Physical Education and Sport. Authors' Contribution: A – Study Design B – Data Collection C – Statistical Analysis D – Manuscript Preparation E – Funds Collection. *Physical Activity Review*. 2. 31–36.

9. Garipagaoglu, M., Budak, N., Süt, N., Akdikmen, O., Oner, N., & Bundak, R. (2009). Obesity Risk Factors in Turkish Children. *Journal of Pediatric Nursing*, 24(4), 332–337. doi: 10.1016/j.pedn.2008.04.003

10. Tremblay, M. S., Leblanc, A. G., Janssen, I., Kho, M. E., Hicks, A., Murumets, K., Colley, R. C. & Duggan, M. (2011). Canadian Sedentary Behaviour Guidelines for Children and Youth. *Appl Physiol Nutr Metab*, 36(1), 59–64. doi: 10.1139/H11-01

11. Simon, C., Schweitzer, B., Oujaa, M., Wagner, A., Arveiler, D., Triby, E., Copin, N., Blanc, S. & Platat, C. (2008). Successful Overweight Prevention in Adolescents by Increasing Physical Activity: A 4-Year Randomized Controlled Intervention. *Int J Obes (Lond)*, 32(10), 1489–1498. doi: 10.1038/ijo.2008.99

12. Physical Activity Review Group. *Five Year Review of 'Let's Make Scotland More Active: A Strategy for Physical Activity': Update Statement from the Review Group*. Edinburgh: NHS Health Scotland, 2010.

13. Corder, K., Sharp, S. J., Atkin, A. J., Griffin, S. J., Jones, A. P., Ekelund, U. & van Sluijs, E. M. (2015). Change in Objectively Measured Physical Activity during the Transition to Adolescence. *Br J Sports Med*, 49(11), 730–736. doi: 10.1136/bjsports-2013-093190

14. Aksoydan, E. & Çakır, N. (2011). Adölesanların beslenme alışkanlıkları, fiziksel aktivite düzeyleri ve vücut kitle indekslerinin değerlendirilmesi. *Gülhane Tıp Dergisi*, 53(4), 264–270.

15. Akman, M., Tüzün, S. & Ünalan, P. C. (2012). Adolesanlarda Sağlıklı Beslenme ve Fiziksel Aktivite Durumu. *Nobel Med*, 8(1), 24–29.

16. Aktürk, S., Büyükavcı, R., & Aktürk, Ü. (2018). Relationship between Musculoskeletal Disorders and Physical Inactivity in Adolescents. *Journal of Public Health*, 1–8. doi: 10.1007/s10389-018-0923-7

17. Inal H.S. *Spor ve Egzersizde Biyomekanik. Temel Prensipler.* Hipokrat Yayınevi. 3rd ed. 2017, Ankara.

18. Magee, D. J., (1987). *Orthopedic Physical Assessment. Gait Assessment.* Toronto: W.B. Saunders Company, Chapter 13, 362–376.

19. Arnold, C. M., Beatty, B., Harrison, E., & Olszynski, W. (2000). The Reliability of Five Clinical Postural Alignment Measures for Women with Osteoporosis. *Physiotherapy Canada*, 52, 287–294.

20. Taft, E. & Frances, R. (2003). Evaluation and Management of Scoliosis. *J Pediatr Health Care*, 17, 42–44. doi:10.1067/mph.2003.7

21. Hedge, A., Morimoto, S. & McCrobie, D. (1999). Effects of Keyboard Tray Geometry on Upper Body Posture and Comfort. *Ergonomics*, 42 (10), 1333–1349. doi: 10.1080/001401399184983

22. Erdinç, O., Hot, K. & Özkaya, M. (2011). Turkish Version of the Cornell Musculoskeletal Discomfort Questionnaire: Cross-Cultural Adaptation and Validation. *Work*, 39 (3), 251–260. doi: 10.3233/WOR-2011-1173

23. Öztürk, M. (2005). *Üniversitede Eğitim-Öğretim Gören Öğrencilerde Uluslararası Fiziksel Aktivite Anketinin Geçerliliği Ve Güvenirliği Ve Fiziksel Aktivite Düzeylerinin Belirlenmesi* (Yüksek Lisans Tezi). Ankara: Hacettepe Üniversitesi Sağlık Bilimleri Enstitüsü.

24. Craig, C. L., Marshall, A. L., Sjöström, M., Bauman, A. E., Booth, M. L., Ainsworth, B. E., Pratt, M., Ekelund, U., Yngve, A., Sallis, J. F. & Oja, P. (2003). International Physical Activity Questionnaire: 12-Country Reliability and Validity. *Medicine & Science in Sports & Exercise*, 35 (8), 1381–1395. doi: 10.1249/01.MSS.0000078924.61453.FB

25. Tekgül, N., Dirik, N., Karademirci, E. & Doğan, A. (2012). Adolesanlarda vücut kitle indeksi (VKİ) ile ilişkili değişkenlerin incelenmesi. *Ege Tıp Dergisi*, 51(3), 183–186.

26. Grimmer, K. A., Williams, M. T. & Gill, T. K. (1999). The Associations between Adolescent Head-on-Neck Posture, Backpack Weight, and Anthropometric Features. *Spine*, 24(21), 2262–2267. doi: 10.1097/00007632-199911010-00015

27. Sur, H., Kolotourou, M., Dimitriou, M., Kocaoglu, B., Keskin, Y., Hayran, O. & Manios, Y. (2005). Biochemical and Behavioral Indices Related to BMI in Schoolchildren in Urban Turkey. *Preventive Medicine*, 41 (2), 614–621. doi: 10.1016/j.ypmed.2004.11.029

40 Gonca Ulker Poschl et al.

28. Vadiveloo, M., Zhu, L. & Quatromoni, P. A. (2009). Diet and Physical Activity Patterns of School-Aged Children. *J Am Diet Assoc*, 109(1), 145–151. doi: 10.1016/j.jada.2008.10.012

29. Ozdirenç, M., Ozcan, A., Akin, F. & Gelecek, N. (2005). Physical Fitness in Rural Children Compared with Urban Children in Turkey. *Pediatrics International*, 47(1), 26–31. doi: 10.1111/j.1442-200x.2004.02008.x

30. Maciałczyk-Paprocka, K., Stawińska-Witoszyńska, B., Kotwicki, T., Sowińska, A., Krzyżaniak, A., Walkowiak, J. & Krzywińska-Wiewiorowska M. (2017). Prevalence of Incorrect Body Posture in Children and Adolescents with Overweight and Obesity. *Eur J Pediatr*, 176, 563–572. doi: 10.1007/s00431-017-2873-4

31. Martínez-Nova, A., Gijón-Noguerón, G., Alfageme-García, P., Montes-Alguacil, J. & Evans, A. M. (2018). Foot Posture Development in Children Aged 5 to11 Years: A Three-Year Prospective Study. *Gait & Posture*, 62, 280–284. doi: 10.1016/j.gaitpost.2018.03.032

32. Gaikwad, P. V. & Ganvir, S. D. (2017). Prevalence of Flat Feet in School Going Boys and Girls in Ahmednagar District. *Paripex - Indian Journal of Research*, 6(7), 21–22. doi: 10.15373/22501991

33. Kang, J. H., Park, R. Y., Lee, S. J., Kim, J. Y., Yoon, S. R., Jung, K. I. (2012). The Effect of the Forward Head Posture on Postural Balance in Long Time Computer Based Worker. *Ann Rehabil Med*, 36(1), 98–104. doi: 10.5535/arm.2012.36.1.98

34. Moore, M. K. (2004). Upper Crossed Syndrome and Its Relationship to Cervicogenic Headache. *Journal of Manipulative and Physiological Therapeutics*, 27(6), 414–420. doi: 10.1016/j.jmpt.2004.05.007

35. Griegel-Morris, P., Larson, K., Mueller-Klaus, K. & Oatis, C. A. (1992). Incidence of Common Postural Abnormalities in the Cervical, Shoulder, and Thoracic Regions and Their Association with Pain in Two Age Groups of Healthy Subjects. *Phys Ther*, 72(6), 425–431.

36. Deveci, S. E., Açık, Y., Gülbayrak, C., Demir, A. F., Karadağ, M. & Koçdemir, E. (2007). İlköğretim öğrencilerinin cep telefonu, bilgisayar, televizyon gibi elektromanyetik alan oluşturan cihazları kullanım sıklığı. *Fırat Tıp Dergisi*, 12(4), 279–283.

37. Straker, L. M., O'Sullivan, P. B., Smith, A. & Perry, M. (2007). Computer Use and Habitual Spinal Posture in Australian Adolescents. *Public Health Rep*, 122(5), 634–643. doi: 10.1177/003335490712200511

Hazal Öksüz and Esra Atılgan

Efficiency of Electromyography Biofeedback with Relaxation Training on Muscle Activation, Disability, and Posture in Chronic Neck Pain

Abstract: *Purpose:* The aim of this study was to compare the effect of classical physiotherapy program in patients with chronic neck pain, in addition to relaxation training with electromyography biofeedback (EMG-BF) on muscle activation level, posture, and disability levels.

Methods: In addition to classical physiotherapy program (Transcutaneous Electrical Nerve Stimulation, ultrasound, hotpack, and home exercise), Group 1 (n = 20, 17 females, 3 males, mean age= 44.85 ± 12.51) was treated with relaxation training with EMG-BF and only classical physiotherapy program was applied to Group 2 (n = 20, 15 female, 5 male, mean age = 43.84 ± 12.33). The treatment applied five days a week for four weeks. Visual Analogue Scale (VAS), goniometric measurements, superficial EMG-BF, Neck Pain and Disability Index (NPDI), and New York Posture Scale (NPS) were used to measure the activation levels of upper trapezius muscle before and after treatment.

Results: In the muscle activation level, there was a significant improvement on the left trapezius in both groups (p=0.005), but in the first group only the right trapezius muscle showed improvement (p=0.003). There was a significant decrease in the scores of NPDI (p=0.012) and NPS (p=0.001).

Conclusion: After treatment, improvement was seen in both groups, but EMG-BF group was found to be more effective in muscle activation, disability, and posture level. It has been concluded that the relaxation training with EMG-BF will provide more effective treatment results by adding classical physiotherapy programs in clinics.

Keywords: Biofeedback, Electromyography, Neck Pain, Rehabilitation, Relaxation, Trapezius

Introduction

Chronic neck pain is an important health problem in modern societies. Nowadays, this problem is frequently encountered. It is the second most common cause of chronic pain after chronic low back pain (1). Approximately 10 % of the adult population has neck pain in at least one period of their lives (2). Many factors in daily living activities cause pain. Physical stresses, static posture, sleep habits, wrong, weight transport, and muscle imbalance are important factors of neck pain (3).

The main reason of muscle imbalance is the loss of endurance in the deep flexor and extensor muscles (4). Accordingly, Type 1 and Type 2 muscle fibers decrease, proprioception gets lost, and, consequently, dysfunction develops (5). In order to compensate for this, an increase activity in the sternocleidomastoid, scalenus anterior, and trapezius muscles of superficial muscles is observed (6). Trapezius muscle, which was the most superficial posterior muscle, is reported that neck pain increased in parallel with the tenderness (7). For this reason, the trapezius muscle is an important place in neck rehabilitation. Data from cervical muscles are important for evaluation, treatment, and rehabilitation.

Biofeedback is the technique of providing biological information to patients in real time that would otherwise be unknown. The most widely used biofeedback among physiotherapists is EMG-BF (8). EMG-BF is a method of retraining muscle by creating new feedback systems as a result of the conversion of myoelectrical signals in the muscle into visual and auditory signals. Thus the patient is self-made to relaxation training (9).

Effective treatment is also provided with active participation of the patient. In the selection of treatment, stretching exercises are often used for trapezius, while relaxation training is often neglected. EMG-BF can be applied in relaxation training with different muscle groups. (10,11).

In studies related to trapezius muscle and EMG-BF, except for neck pain, it was also used in scapular dysfunction, shoulder problems, temporomandibular dysfunction, and headache (12,13). There are also studies investigating the relationship between trapezius muscle and neck pain and providing relaxation training with EMG-BF (14,15). However, EMG-BF training was designed in patients with neck pain, because of lack of adequate study comparing activity limitation and posture.

Method and Material

This descriptive study was conducted in Physical Therapy and Rehabilitation Clinic, Istanbul Medipol University Health Application Center, Sefaköy Hospital.

Inclusion and Exclusion Criteria

Patients with chronic neck pain between 18 and 65 years of age were included in the study. Patients with neurological problems, visual hearing loss, cervical region-related surgery, cervical region tumors and infections, cervical steroid injections in the last 3 months were not included in the study.

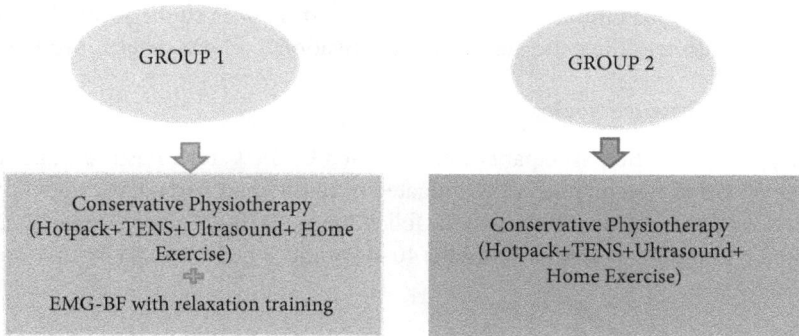

Fig. 1: Conservative physiotherapy and EMG-BF group

Forty-one individuals were divided into two groups as conservative physiotherapy with EMG-BF and the second group as conservative physiotherapy randomly. The groups were separated by simple randomization method (heads and tails).

In the first group, conservative physiotherapy consisted of ultrasound, TENS, hotpack and home exercise, relaxation training with EMG-BF (Group 1) and random conservative physiotherapy were applied to the second group (Group 2).

Ethics Committee Approval

Our study was evaluated at Istanbul Medipol University Non-invasive Clinical Research Ethics Committee meeting on 28.10.2015 and it was approved by file number 10840098–604.01.01-E.3201. *The patients who were included in the study were informed about the study and signed their consent.*

Data Collection Method and Instruments

A form to record the socio-demographic characteristics of the cases was prepared. In this assessment, various factors including age, height, body weight, BMI, were considered.

EMG-BF

EMG-BF (Intelect Advanced Color Combo + EMG, Chattanooga Group, TN, USA) was used to evaluate muscle activation level. The screen scale was used as a visual feedback, as an increased or decreasing signal tone with varying muscle activity as sensory feedback. Before the treatment, the target was determined.

Ten seconds of maximum contraction and relaxation were studied with the "Set Target" on device. Thus, the mean muscle activation level was determined (16).

New York Posture Scale

The postures of the participants were assessed by New York Posture Scale. In this evaluation system, posture is evaluated in 13 different parts of the body. The scores are interpreted according to the following guide: 0–19 points = bad; 20–29 points = weak; 30–39 points = middle; 40–44 points = good; and 45 point = very good (17).

Neck Pain and Disability Scale

Disability was assessed by Neck Pain and Disability Scale. Reliability and validity of its Turkish version was tested by Biçer et al. It evaluates the severity of pain and its effect on occupational, recreational, social, daily living activities and the relationship with emotional factors. Neck Pain and Disability Scale consists of 20 items. Scoring is made between 0 and 5 points. High scores indicate more severe pain and affect (18).

Treatment Program

In Group 1, EMG-BF was applied in addition to conservative physiotherapy program. In Group 2, only conservative physiotherapy was applied. Treatment was planned as 20 sessions to be performed on 5 days per week for 4 weeks. The participants in both groups received home exercise program. The exercise program involved strengthening exercises and ROM exercises including neck flexion, extension, right/left lateral flexion along with stretching exercises for upper trapezius, posterior part of deltoid, and pectoral muscles to be practiced three times a day with ten repetitions. EMG-BF training should be performed on 5 days per week for 4 weeks. Upper and middle trapezius relaxation training was performed as 20 repetitions for 5 seconds maximum contract and 10 seconds for rest. During training, the device screen is placed where the patients can see. The values in the device are shown in the vertical graph in microvolts. The education is continued by aiming the patient to fall below the predetermined mean value. The device is a Chattanoga Group Intelect Advanced Color Combo + EMG.

Statistical Analysis

All analyses were performed with the SPSS (version 22.0) statistical package program. The level of significance was set at $p < 0.05$. Data were evaluated using descriptive statistics (number, percentage, distribution, average, and standard deviation). Kolmogorov-Smirnov method was used for evaluation of normal distribution. A paired t-test was used to compare pre- and post-treatment results of each group. An independent t-test was used to determine the changes in the experimental group compared to the control group (reported as the mean±standard deviation). The statistical significance level was set at $p < 0.05$.

Results

A total of 40 patients with chronic neck pain were included in the study. Demographic variables of the participants are provided in Tab. 1. No statistical difference was found between the groups regarding demographic data (gender, age, job, and diagnoses).

Muscle activations were analyzed by surface EMG. A significant change was observed in both groups on the right side (p=0,005) after treatment and only a significant change was observed on the left side in Group 1 (p=0,003). The upper trapezius EMG results are shown in Tab. 2.

In the second group there were development unprecedented in neck pain and disability index, but there was a favorable change in the first group. In the New York Posture Scale, scores were increased in both groups after treatment, but the improvement was more significant in the first group (p = 0.02). The results of postural assessment were given in Tab. 3.

Discussion

The prevalence of neck pain is 30–50 % in adults (19). These individuals usually receive conservative physiotherapy in clinics. There isn't use of exercise or

Tab. 1: Socio-Demographic Information of Individuals

	Group1 n=20)		Group 2 n=20		p
Woman	N	%	n	%	0,442*
Man	17	85	15	75	
	3	15	5	25	
Age (year)	44,85 ±12,51		43,84±12,33		0,605*
BMI (kg/m²)	28,18±12,33		29,68± 12,51		0,403*

* Independent t-test was used p<0.05.
BMI: Body Mass Index

Tab. 2: Upper Trapezius EMG Value

	Right Upper Trapezius EMG value			Intergroup comparison P	Left Upper Trapezius EMG value			Intergroup comparison P
	BT	AT	p		BT	AT	p	
Group 1	35,50±21,2	21,55±3,53	0,00*	0,005*	32,45±3,53	21,36±12,1	0,00*	0,003*
Group 2	27,35±19,7	22,7±15,55	0,025*		30,20±10,61	26,80±2,12	0,14*	

* Independent t-test was used p<0.05.
BT: Before Treatment, AT: After Treatment

Tab. 3: Neck Pain and Disability Index vs New York Posture Scale Intergroup Comparison Before and After Treatment

	Before treatment	After treatment	p	Intergroup comparison p
Neck Pain and Disability Index Group 1 Group 2	51,30±28,28 48,95±13,43	17,21±9,17 40,25±34,64	0,00* 0,088*	0,00*
New york Posture Scale Group 1 Group 2	45,75±16,97 52,50±5,65	56,75±0,00 54,9±6,19	0,00* 0,012*	0,002*

* Independent t-test was used, p<0.05

rehabilitation protocol for neck rehabilitation (20). Conservative physiotherapy has a healing effect on neck patients, but the efficacy of treatment is insufficient.

The biomechanical and psychosocial causes of musculoskeletal problems in working individuals were investigated. For the measurement of muscle activation, the relationship between trapezius muscle and neck pain is emphasized by using EMG. Thus, the trapezius muscle was closely associated with neck and shoulder problems (21). Studies have shown a connection between upper trapezius muscle activation and neck problems (22; 23). In the review, EMG-BF applied in neck pain was reported to be effective in reducing symptoms (23). Yang and collegues (2017) were determined that muscle activity values and tonus decreased while relaxation levels decreased (24). Our study was performed by adding relaxation training with EMG-BF to upper trapezius muscle in addition to conservative physiotherapy. We expect a reduction in disability due to a decrease in muscle activation values.

Our study was performed by adding relaxation training with EMG-BF to upper trapezius muscle in addition to conservative physiotherapy. We expect a reduction in disability due to a decrease in muscle activation values. Apelyan (2012) has examined trapezius muscle spasm pain in chronic pain neck sendrome. The study included 34 individuals and they were separated into two groups. EMG-BF relaxation training was applied to the intervention group and hot pack and TENS were applied to the control group. Both groups were treated with 10 sessions and were given isometric training as a home program (25). VAS and joint motion measurements were performed before and after the treatment. After the treatment, both groups had decreased pain and increased range of motion, but there wasn't difference between the group (26).In our study, in order to prevent the expected effect on neck pain, conservative physiotherapy program was added to both groups. The results of the treatments were also favourable. Thus, the results in the EMG-BF group were more contented.

As neck pain increases, it causes muscle fatigue. Disability was also increased due to increased muscle fatigue (27). Previous investigation focused on effect of treatment of the patients with neck pain on the limitation of the activity by using EMG-BF. As a result of the study, EMG-BF applied muscle relaxation and decrease in pain. In our study, NPDI results showed a significant improvement in both groups, but the results were more effective in the EMG-BF group. We think that because the treatment program includes classical physiotherapy and EMG-BF training, the patient is more likely to recover from relaxation (28).

Posture is the position of every part of the body in the most suitable position relative to the whole body and the segment adjacent to it. Studies have reported poor posture, anxiety, depression, and quality of life problems in patients with chronic neck pain (29). Gaffney and colleagues (2015) were measuring EMG on the trapezius muscle, there was a correlation between body posture and EMG values (30).

At different body positions, the EMG and muscle activation values of the upper trapezius were examined. The muscle activation level in the neutral posture was found to be the lowest (31). Newyork Posture Scale was used to evaluate posture of individuals in our study. Significant improvement was observed in both groups after the treatment. But the results are more significant effect than the results of the first group.

EMG-BF increased the awareness of posture. There was a favorable change in all measurement parameters of EMG-BF Groups. It is seen that conservative treatment is an effective treatment in patients with chronic neck pain, but more effective treatment results will be obtained by EMG-BF administration under the supervision of physiotherapist in relaxation training.

Limitations

There are some limitations that need to be acknowledged. In our study, the short term effects of the treatment were evaluated in four weeks. Future studies are required to investigate long-term effect EMG-BF training in chronic neck pain. Individuals were recruited into two groups. However, the comparison could be more effective if there was third group and can only be treated with EMG-BF without conservative physiotherapy.

Disclosure Statement

We would like to state that the above-mentioned manuscript has not been published elsewhere, has not been accepted for publication elsewhere, or under editorial review for publication elsewhere.

Conflict of Interest

There is no conflict of interest by the authors. This study has not been published anywhere before.

Financial Disclosure

The authors declared that they did not receive any financial support for this study

References

1. Tunwattanapong P, Kongkasuwan R, Kuptniratsaikul V. (2016) The Effectiveness of a Neck and Shoulder Stretching Exercise Program among Office Workers with Neck Pain: A Randomized Controlled Trial. *Clin Rehabil.*; 30(1):64–72.

2. Bruflat AK, Balter JE, McGuire D, Fethke NB, Maluf KS (2012) Stress Management as an Adjunct to Physical Therapy for Chronic Neck Pain. *Phys Ther.*; 10, 1348–59.

3. Şengül YS. (2014) Bel boyun problemlerinde fizyoterapi. In: Algun C. (Ed) *Fizik Tedavi ve Rehabilitasyon*. İstanbul, Nobel Tıp Kitapevi; p. 271–287.

4. Tsang SMH., SO BCL, Lau RW.L, Dai J. (2018) Effects of Combining Ergonomic Interventions and Motor Control Exercises on Muscle Activity and Kinematics in People with Work Related Neck–Shoulder Pain. *Eur J Appl Physiol.*; 118(4):751-765.

5. Falla D, Farina D, Jull G. (2011) Association Between Intensity of Pain and Impairment in Onset and Activation of the Deep Cervical Flexors in Patients

with Persistent Neck Pain. *Clin J Pain*; 27(4):309–14.

6. Fernández-de-las-Peñas C, Alonso-Blanco C, Miangolarra JC. (2007) Myofascial Trigger Points in Subjects Presenting with Mechanical Neck Pain: A Blinded, Controlled Study. *Man Ther.*; 12(1):29–33.

7. Brandt M, Sundstrup E, Jakobsen MD, Jay K, Colado JC, Wang Y. (2014) Association between Neck/Shoulder Pain and Trapezius Muscle Tenderness in Office Workers. *Pain Research and Treatment*; 2090–1550.

8. Giggins OM, Persson UM, Caulfield B. (2013) Biofeedback in Rehabilitation. *J Neuroeng Rehabil. Bio Med Central*; 18; 10(1):60.

9. Basmajian J V. (1988) Research Foundations of EMG Biofeedback in Rehabilitation. *Biofeedback and Self-Regulation*; 13(4):275–98.

10. Baumueller E, Winkelmann A, Irnich D, Weigl M. (2017) Electromyogram Biofeedback in Patients with Fibromyalgia: A Randomized Controlled Trial. *Complement Med Res.* 24(1):33–39.

11. Crider A, Glaros G. (1999) A Meta-Analysis of EMG Biofeedback Treatment of Temporomandibular Disorders. *Journal of Orofarangial Pain.*; 29–38.

12. Castelein B, Cools A, Bostyn E, Delemarre J, Lemahieu T, Cagnie B. (2015) Analysis of Scapular Muscle EMG Activity in Patients with Idiopathic Neck Pain : A Systematic Review. *J Electromyogr Kinesiol.*; 25(2):371–86.

13. Tali D, Menahem I, Vered E, Kalichman L. (2014) Upper Cervical Mobility, Posture and Myofascial Trigger Points in Subjects with Episodic Migraine: Case-Control Study. *J Bodyw Mov Ther.*; 18(4):569–75.

14. Tsang SMH, So BCL, Lau RWL, Dai J, Szeto GPY. (2018) Effects of Combining Ergonomic Interventions and Motor Control Exercises on Muscle Activity and Kinematics in People with Work Related Neck–Shoulder Pain. *Eur J Appl Physiol.*; 118(4):751-765.

15. Blödt S, Pach D, Roll S, Witt CM. (2014) Effectiveness of App-Based Relaxation for Patients with Chronic Low Back Pain and Chronic Neck Pain: Study Protocol for Two Randomized Pragmatic Trials. *Trials*; 15–490.

16. Belanger AY. (2008) *Kanıta Dayalı Elektroterapi*, p. 217–220 1. T. Yakut E, Dlkılıç M, Kaya D. Pelikan Yayınları, Ankara.

17. Mcroberts LB, Cloud RM, Black CM. (2013) Evaluation of the New York Posture Rating Chart for Assessing Changes in Postural Alignment in a Garment Study. *Clothing and Textiles Research Journal*; 31(2), 81–96.

18. Bicer A, Yazici A, Camdeviren H, Erdogan C. (2004) Assessment of Pain and Disability in Patients with Chronic Neck Pain: Reliability and Construct Validity of the Turkish Version of the Neck Pain and Disability Scale. *Disabil Rehabil.*; 26(16):959–62.

19. Fejer R, Hartvigsen J. (2008) Neck Pain and Disability due to Neck Pain: What Is the Relation? *Eur Spine J*; 80–8.

20. Ylinen J. (2007) Physical Exercises and Functional Rehabilitation for the Management of Chronic Neck Pain. *Europa Medicophysica.*;43(1):119–32.

21. Westgaard RH. (2000) Work-Related Musculoskeletal Complaints: Some Ergonomics Challenges upon the Start of a New Century. *Appl Ergon.*; 31:569–80.

22. Chaikumarn M, Nakphet N & Janwantanakul P. (2017) Repeatability of Electromyography Normalization of the Neck and Shoulder Muscles in Symptomatic Office Workers. *Int J Occup Saf Ergon.*; 10.1080.

23. Findley JL, Monticone M, Pappas E, Campo M. (2015) Biofeedback for Neck Pain. Biofeedback for Neck Pain. *Cochrane Database of Systematic Reviews*; 10.1002.

24. Yang DJ, Kang DH. (2017) Comparison of Muscular Fatigue and Tone of Neck according to Craniocervical Flexion Exercise and Suboccipital Relaxation in Cervicogenic Headache Patients. *International Journal of Occupational Safety and Ergonomics*; 1080–3548.

25. Apelyan A. (2002) Boyun Ağrılarında Biofeedback ile Kas Gevşetme Eğitiminin Etkinliği. *M.Ü. Sağlık Bilimleri Enstitüsü*, İstanbul.

26. El-Abd AM, Ibrahim AR, El-Hafez HM. (2017) Efficacy of Kinesiology Tape versus Postural Correction Exercises on Neck Disability and Axioscapular Muscles Fatigue in Mechanical Neck Dysfunction: A Randomized Blinded Clinical Trial. *J Bodyw Mov Ther.* 21(2):314–321.

27. Voerman G, Miriam MR. (2007) Changes in Pain, Disability, and Muscle Activation Patterns in Chronic Whiplash Patients after Ambulant Myofeedback Training: Commentary. Headache. *Clin J Pain.* 47(3):458–9.

28. Watson AW, Mac DC. (2000) A Reliable Technique for the Assessment of Posture: Assessment Criteria for Aspects of Posture. *J Sport Med Phys Fit.*; 40:260–70.

29. Heintz M, Hegedus E. (2007) Multimodal Management of Mechanical Neck Pain Using a Treatment Based Classification System. *J Man Ther.* 16(4): 217–24.

30. Gaffney BM, Maluf KS, Davidson BS. (2015) Evaluation of Novel EMG Biofeedback for Postural Correction during Computer Use. *Appl Psychophysiol Biofeedback Springer US*; 10.1007.

31. Gonçalves JS, Shinohara C, Kawa MKST, Coury H. (2017) The Effect of Forearm Support and Shoulder Posture on Upper Trapezius an Anterior Deltoid Activity, *The Journal of Physical Therapy Science*; 29(5): 793–798.

Jülide Öncü Alptekin, Ahmet Üşen, Banu Kuran, and Kerem Alptekin

Changes in Hand Bone Density after Distal Radius Fracture and Correlation with Clinical Parameters: A Longitudinal Study[1]

Abstract: *Study Design:* Prospective, case-control study

Background: Post-fracture loss of bone density has been a well known phenomenon. However, there was a paucity in the literature about changes in hand bone densitometry in patients having distal radius fracture. And also, it's unclear whether there is a relationship between disease parameters.

Objective: To measure hand bone mineral density (BMD) by dual x-ray absorptiometry and to investigate clinical correlates in patients with DRF in a prospective, longitudinal study.

Material and Methods: Forty-nine patients with DRF (21 women, (range 30 to 43 years); 28 men (range 30 to 56 years)) were included in the study. Patients were divided into 2 groups according to having diagnosed of CRPS: Group I: Patients with CRPS (DRF/CRPS); Group II: Patients without CRPS (DRF/non-CRPS). All tests were undertaken at the 1st visit at the time when the patient came to our clinic and at the 2nd visit (52nd week).

Results: The group-analysis showed that in group I (DRF/CRPS) hand BMD of fractured side (t score: -2.5) was found to be statistically lower than those of group II (DRF/non-CRPS) (t score: -1.2) at the 2nd visit (p<0.05). Within the group analysis, a statistically significant decrease in fractured hand BMD has been found during one year, only in Group I (p<0.05) (t score from -1.3 to -2.5). Correlation analysis showed that the clinical parameters at the 1st visit were significantly negatively correlated with the hand BMD of the 2nd visit only in group I (DRF/CRPS) (SHSS: r=-0.209, p=0.008; DASH: r=-0.120, p=0.01; VAS: r=-0.149; p=0.031). There was no correlation between hand BMD and other clinical and demographical indices (p>0.05).

Conclusion: These results showed that there was a significant reduction of hand BMD in patients with distal radius fracture with CRPS during one year. The reduction in BMD correlated with the severity of CRPS, pain, and upper extremity dysfunction.

Keywords: Densitometry, Radius, Fracture, Osteoporosis

---

1   This manuscript was accepted as poster presentation at National Physical Medicine and Rehabilitation Congress 2015.

Introduction

Post-fracture loss of bone density has been a well known phenomenon (1). It's so-called regional osteoporosis, which is distal to the fracture site and associated with increased bone turnover (2). Studies investigating the regional osteoporosis showed that extremity fractures were associated with persistent post-traumatic loss of distal bone mineral density (BMD) leaving the patients vulnerable to the second fracture (1–3). Regional osteoporosis was studied mostly after lower extremity fractures by dual energy X-Ray absorptiometry (DEXA) (3,4). It has been found that in patients with tibial fracture, there was a significant decrement in BMD, which was detected by ankle and foot DEXA (1,3,4). Although these findings are well-established after lower extremity fractures, some attention has been raised recently with respect to the hand osteoporosis after distal radius fractures (DRF) and very little longitudinal evidence is available regarding regional hand bone loss secondary to DRF. DRF are the most common upper extremity fracture (5). It occurs in a bimodal distribution with the highest frequency in younger patients without osteoporosis who sustain athletic and high-energy trauma and a second peak in older patients with osteoporosis (5). DRF were often associated with a poor outcome because an overall complication rate has been reported as 31 %including neuropathies, tendon ruptures, contractures, and Complex Regional Pain Syndrome (CRPS) (6). An incidence of CRPS can rise up to 37 % after DRF (7). Therefore DRF and its complications, especially CRPS, result in significant disability, reduced quality of life, and substantial economic burden to health systems worldwide (7). CRPS is a debilitating condition affecting the limbs that is characterised by severe pain along with sensory, autonomic, motor, trophic impairment, and regional osteoporosis (6,7). Fractures appear to be a common inciting event for the development of CRPS; especially more common evidence is present in upper extremity in contrast to lower extremity in the literature (8). Region-specific osteoporosis, which is characterized by elevated bone turnover and bone resorptions, is one of the comorbidities of CRPS; however, there is lack of published data on this topic, especially after DRF (8). Up to date, the information about the rate of hand bone loss after DRF and its time course is very limited, and also the clinical parameters including CRPS have not been investigated yet. Considering these findings, the aim of our study was to investigate the hand bone loss after DRF and also to investigate the effect of clinical parameters including CRPS during one year in a longitudinal design.

Material and Methods

Objective

To measure hand bone mineral density (BMD) by dual x-ray absorptiometry and to investigate clinical correlates in patients with DRF, in a prospective, longitudinal study.

The Universe and Sample of Research

Subjects

Forty-nine patients with DRF (21 women, range 30 to 43 years); 28 men (range 30 to 56 years) were included into the study.

Inclusion and Exclusion Criteria

Patients with DRF after high-energy trauma who were referred to our clinic for rehabilitation were selected for this study. Patients who had closed, nondisplaced, and unilateral distal radius fractures were treated conservatively and who had intellectual capacity to give informed consent for participation were included. Patients who were unwilling or unable to participate (due to insufficient cognitive functioning) had surgically treated DRF, had osteoporotic fractures, had already diagnosed with primary and secondary osteoporosis (inflammatory arthritis, hyperparathyroidism, thyroid dysfunction, metabolic bone diseases, and renal dysfunction), had bilateral fracture, had intra-articular or unstable DRF, and had fractures due to malignancy were excluded.

Data Collection Tools and Data Collection

Personal Information Form

Demographical characteristics regarding gender, age, weight, height, body mass index (BMI:kg/m2), dominant hand side, fractured site, and educational level were recorded. (fig 1)

Measurements

Hand grip strength was measured by using a dynamometer (baseline hydraulic hand dynamometer, Irvington, NY, USA) defined by American Hand Therapists Association (9). The measurements were taken three times, and the value of hand grip strength was determined as the average of the best results of these 3 trials (9,10). All participants were examined in a standardized position (10). *The range of motion of the wrist* (flexion, extension, pronation, supination, and ulnar and radial deviation) was evaluated by a standard goniometer and reported in degrees (11).

For diagnosis of CRPS, "The Budapest Criteria" were used to discriminate the subjects having symptoms of CRPS (12). Patients were divided into 2 groups according to having diagnosis of CRPS: Group I: Patients with CRPS (DRF/CRPS); Group II: Patients without CRPS (DRF/non-CRPS).

Laboratory analysis were taken before the study (serum calcium, phosphorus, alkaline phosphatase, parathyroid hormone, thyroid and renal function tests, and, also, acute phase reactants) to exclude any other disease causing osteoporosis (inflammatory arthritis, hyperparathyroidism, thyroid dysfunction, metabolic bone diseases, and renal dysfunction).

Dual Energy X-Ray Absorptiometry (DEXA)

All patients underwent BMD measurement of the fractured and contralateral (normal) hand by dual energy X-ray absorptiometry (DEXA) using a Lunar Prodigy Advance DEXA. For whole hand DEXA, all hand bones distal from the wrist joint were included in the measurement, as described by Deodhar et al. (13); the hand flat on a table and the fingers extended. The entire hand was scanned and a bone map was created. BMD was calculated in gram/cm^2 (13,14) (Fig. 1).

All patients were evaluated by lumbar and hip DEXA to exclude currently existing general osteoporosis.

Shoulder Hand Syndrome Score (SHSS)

The shoulder hand syndrome score (SHSS) was used to grade the severity of CRPS-I (15,16) It has been used to examine CRPS, and it measures the severity of clinical symptoms (pain and hyperalgesia, distal oedema, painless range of motion). The total score of SHS ranges from 0 (none) to 14 (the most severe) (16).

Disability of Arm Shoulder Hand Questionnaire (DASH)

For the disability of arm shoulder hand (DASH) score, a self-administrated questionnaire, which includes 30 items related to functional activities and symptoms in activities of daily living (ADL), was used. The patients were asked to attribute a score of 1 to 5 on all 30 items (17). Scores rise with increasing disability (17). The values are summed and divided by the number of questions answered. This value is transformed to a score out of 100 by subtracting 1 and multiplying by 25.

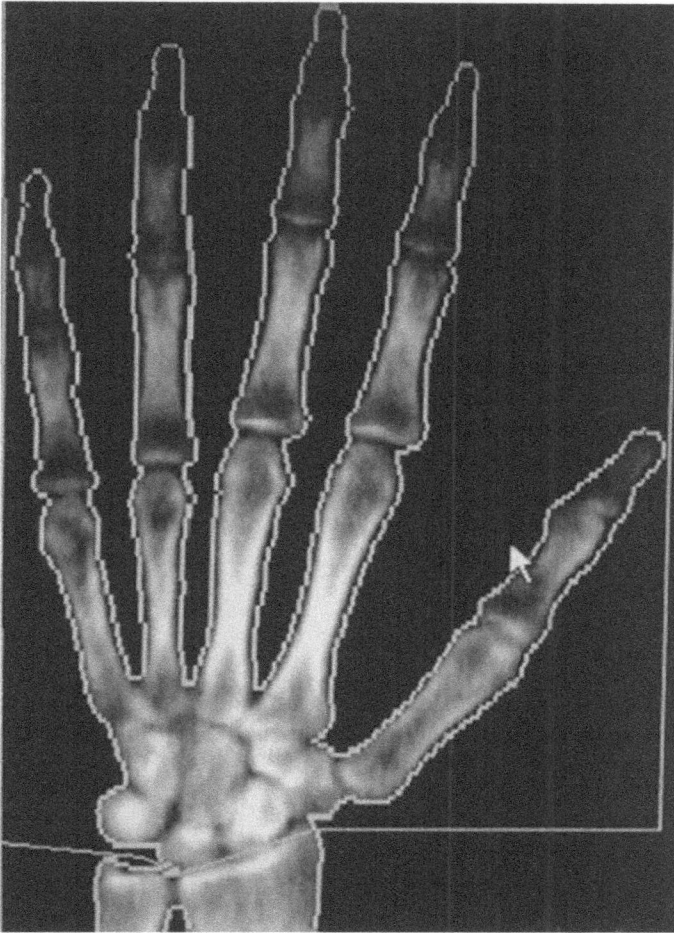

Fig. 1: Hand Bone Densitometry Measurement Region of İnterest of the Hand of Study Subjects

Pain Severity

To assess pain intensity, subjects were asked to rate their average pain over the past 24 hours on a 10-cm visual analog scale (VAS) ranging from 0 cm (indicating no pain) to 10 cm (indicating pain as bad as you can imagine). Higher scores indicate greater pain severity (18).

Visits

Patients were referred to our clinic from orthopedics after the callus formation at the 8th week of the fracture (1st visit). All tests were undertaken at the 1st visit at the time when the patient came to our clinic and at the 2nd visit (one year after 1st visit).

Statistical Analysis

Descriptive statistics were reported for continuous variables using mean and standard deviations (SDs) and for categorical variables using counts. Before performing the analyses, the normality of the distribution of the data was evaluated using the one-sample Kolmogorov-Smirnov test. This test indicated that the data had non-normal distribution (z:0.503, p:0.0438). For the correlation of the clinical and densitometric results, Spearman correlation coefficients were determined. Wilcoxon signed rank test was used to test the mean differences in the outcomes between the two visits. Kruskal Wallis test was used for the multiple group comparisons. SPSS-17.0 was used for the analysis. The alpha level for determining statistical significance was set at 0.05. Power Analysis was not conducted before the study.

Ethical Aspects of Research

Written informed consent was provided by each subject. Our study was approved by the Ethics Committee of Şişli Hamidiye Etfal Training Hospital (04.2011–33).

Results

Similar demographical characteristics were observed between the groups (p>0.05). The characteristics of the patients included in our study are presented in Tab. 1.

The group analysis between the groups showed that in group I (DRF/CRPS), hand BMD of fractured side (t score: -2.5) was found to be statistically lower than those of group II (DRF/non-CRPS) (t score:-1.2) at the 2nd visit (p<0.05) (values for all groups are presented by Fig. 2).

When compared to contralateral normal hands (in both visits, t-score in Group I: +0.0, in Group II: +0.0), hand BMDs of the fractured side were statistically low in both groups (all p values are shown on Fig. 3).

Within the group-analysis, a statistically significant decrease in fractured hand BMD has been found during one year, only in Group I (p<0.05) (Fig. 4) (t score from -1.3 to -2.5).

Tab. 1: Demographic and Clinical Characteristics of the Study Group

	Group I (with CRPS) (n=23)		Group II (without CRPS) (n=26)	
	Mean± SD		Mean± SD	Median(Min,Max)
Age (years)	43.2 ±12.0	43 (28, 56)	43.4 ± 10.5	(30, 55)
Educational status	91.2			91.1
- Low-graduate (high school)(%)	9,2			9.3
- High-graduate (university)(%)				
BMI (kg/m2)	27.3±5.3	27 (19,39)	27.2± 5.1	27 (18,39)
Fractured side (Right-hand)(%)	49.0		50 %	
Dominant hand (Right-hand)(%)	100.0		99.0	
VAS-pain (0–100 mm)	89 ±19	100 (30,100)	2,1± 0,5	2,5(2,3)
SHS score (0–14)	12.3 ± 2.3	11 (7,15)	-	-
DASH score (0–100)	65.5 ± 21.5	64 (38,96)	22,1±9,2	20(10,30)

BMI: body mass index; SD: standard deviation, Min: minimum; Max: maximum; VAS: visual analog scale; SHS: shoulder hand syndrome: DASH: disability of arm shoulder hand

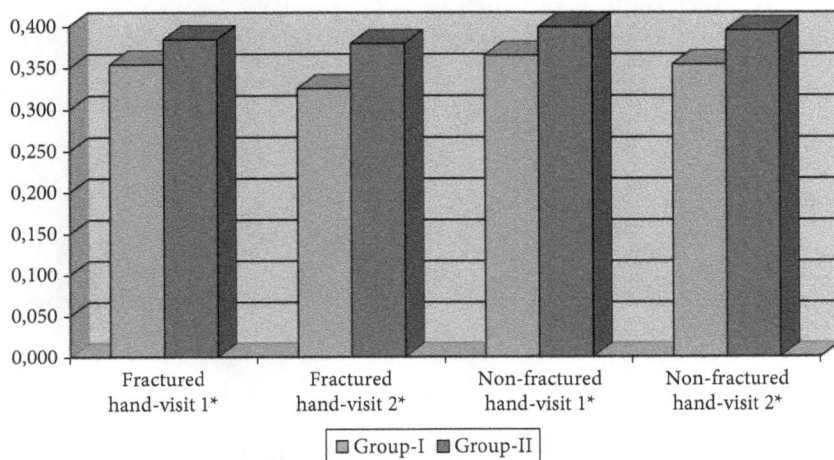

Fig. 2: The Differences of Hand BMDs'(gram/cm^2) between the Groups. Group I: Patients with DRF and CRPS. Group II: Patients with DRF without CRPS. *$p<0.05$

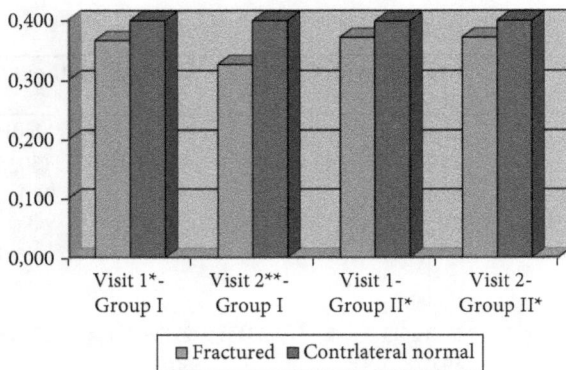

Fig. 3: The Differences of Hand BMDs'(gram/cm2) between the Fractured and Contralateral Normal Hand. Group I: Patients with DRF and CRPS. Group II: Patients with DRF without CRPS. Visit 1: Baseline visit. Visit 2: Visit at the 52th Week *p<0.05**p<0.01

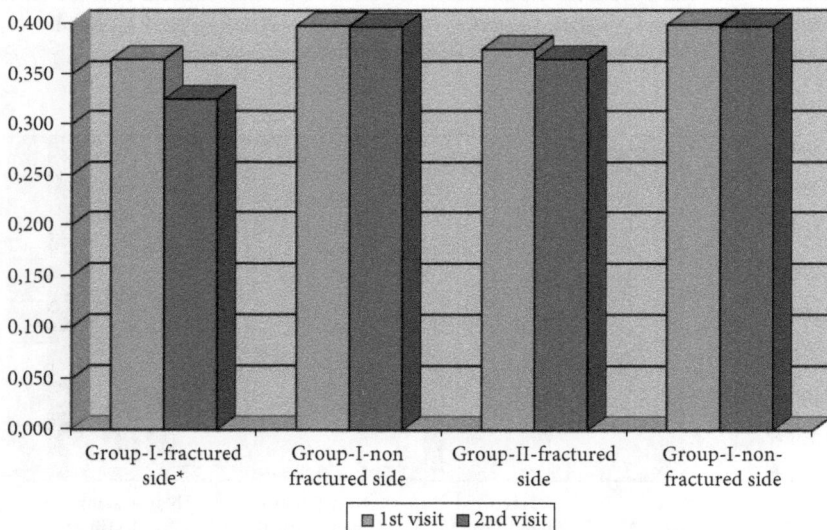

Fig. 4: The Differences in Hand BMDs'(gram/cm^2) within The Groups During One Year. Group I: Patients with DRF and CRPS. Group II: Patients with DRF without CRPS. Visit 1: Baseline Visit. Visit 2: Visit at the 52th Week *p<0.05

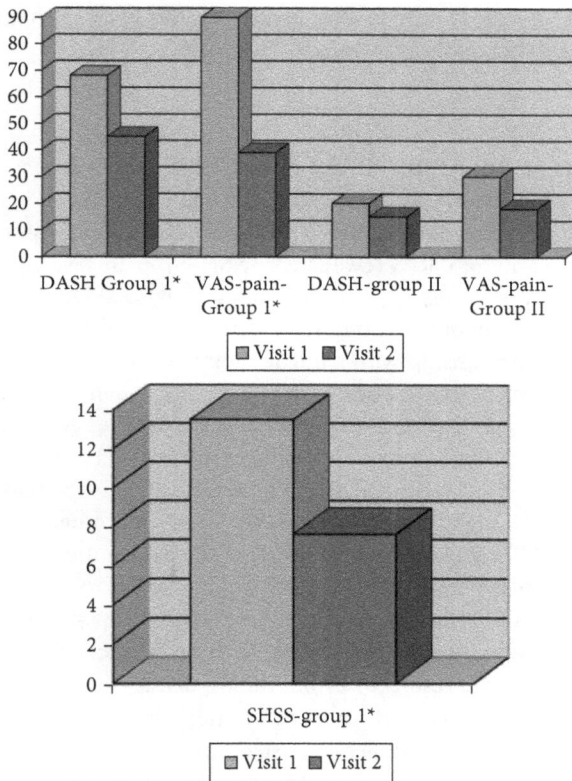

Fig. 5: a) DASH (Disability of Arm Shoulder Hand) and VAS(Visual Analog Scale)-Pain Scores between the Two Visits. Visit 1: Baseline Visit. Visit 2: Visit at the 52th Week *p<0.05. **b)** SHSS: Scores of Shoulder Hand Syndrome. Visit 1: Baseline Visit. Visit 2: Visit at the 52th Week.*p<0.05

Regarding clinical parameters, between the group analysis showed that in Group I, scores of SHS (p<0.05), DASH (p<0.01), and VAS-pain severity (p<0.05) were significantly worse than those of Group II only at baseline visit. The analysis within the group showed that a statistically significant improvement was observed in these parameters only in Group I during one year (Fig. 4). Some improvement has been observed in Group II; however, this was not significant (Fig. 5a–b).

Correlation analysis showed that the clinical parameters at the 1st visit were significantly negatively correlated with the hand BMD of the 2nd visit only in group I (DRF/CRPS) (SHSS: r=-0.209, p=0.008; DASH: r=-0.120, p=0.01;

VAS: r=-0.149; p=0.031). There were no correlation between hand BMD and other clinical and demographical indices (p>0.05).

Discussion

The results of this study provide the novel evidence that when compared to patients without CRPS the patients with CRPS had continued to lose hand bone density during one year after fracture. And this bone loss was significantly related to the initial severity of CRPS (evaluated by SHSS), pain severity according to VAS and dysfunction of the upper limb (evaluated by DASH). There was a paucity in the literature about the long-term course of hand bone loss after wrist fractures and its relationship with clinical parameters (as a whole picture; pain severity, CRPS severity, dysfunction of upper extremity, hand grip strength, etc.). It has been known that general osteoporosis is the alteration of bone microarchitecture due to aging or hormonal dysfunction (19). On the other side, the regional osteoporosis, or localized demineralization, is the bone loss due to immobilisation of skeletal site due to fracture, pain syndrome, or inflammatory erosive diseases (20). Regional osteoporosis of the extremities has been studied mostly in studies of rheumatoid arthritis (RA) (13,14) and to a lesser extent, after extremity fractures (2–4). Until now, there were only a few studies investigating the effect of CRPS on bone loss after lower extremity fractures in the literature (2–4). According to the results of these studies, it was established that it was a defined pathological entity, with causes and etiopathogenetic mechanisms different from those at the base of general osteoporosis (2–4,8). In this study, to be able to monitor the progression of regional osteoporosis alone, we have excluded general osteoporosis at the beginning of the study by means of femur and lumbar DEXA measurements. On this count, we were able to follow regional bone loss after DRF in the hand without interfering with general osteoporosis during one year. And our results showed that although none of our patients had general osteoporosis but all of them had regional bone loss on the fractured side compared to normal contralateral side. Therefore, it is possible to say that DRF results in regional osteoporosis in the hand which is detectable by hand DEXA. This finding is similar to the studies about regional osteoporosis after lower extremity fractures. In order to detect regional hand bone loss, we used DEXA of whole hand as described by Deodhar (13), reflecting primarily phalangeal resorption. It has been used in many of the studies especially in rheumatoid arthritis and reported that it was feasible and had good precision (13,21). It has been found advantageous over lumbar and femur DEXA in early diagnosis of the disease (11,20–22). And it is a sensitive clinical outcome measure to follow-up the effect of treatment (11,20–22). Although the situation has been clearly defined in RA, there is a paucity in the literature about the changes in hand bone loss after DRF. Up to date there is only one clinical trial investigating regional hand bone loss after DRF (2). The authors stated that there was significant loss in hand BMD, which was detectable by hand DEXA (2). In addition, this bone loss was correlated with bone turnover biomarkers and findings of quantitative ultrasound (2). Therefore, it is useful method in follow-up of these kind of patients. Supportingly, our results showed that hand DEXA was useful not only to detect regional osteoporosis at baseline, but also to monitor the loss of hand bone mineral density after DRF during one year. Our study is the second one investigating the hand bone loss after DRF, in a longitudinal design. Ingle et al. (2) investigated the changes in bone mass in the hand and bone turnover following DRF during one year. And the authors reported that a significant regional hand bone loss occured in fractured side (9 %) when compared to normal hand in 6 weeks after DRF. Similarly, our results showed that there was a significant bone loss in fractured side when compared to contralateral hand in both groups at the 1st visit (in 8th weeks of the fracture after the removal of the cast). In patients without CRPS this regional bone loss might be due to the effect of immobilisation under the cast during 8 weeks. And it has been reported that one of the early responses of the immobilisation after fracture is that an increase in bone turnover at distal sites (2,3). In another study investigating bone mineral loss after tibial fracture, this turnover became to evident in one month of the immobilisation and felt to approximately 50 % in three months (3). Additionally Ingle et al.(2) have found that this significant hand bone loss did not recover by 52 weeks, just like our patients without CRPS whose loss of hand BMDs on fractured side remained decreased during one year. According to results of the studies, there was certain amount of bone loss at distal sites after extremity fracture and remained decreased (described as persistant loss) during one or two years (2,3). This is due to the changes in bone remodelling. After immobilisation, there is a good evidence that bone turnover is increased, but the amount of newly formed bone laid down in erosion cavities is less than normal (3,23). The imbalance between formation and resorption gives rise to this persistent bone loss (3,23). In accordance with these findings, in our study, hand BMD in patients without CRPS remained decreased (did not recover) after one year. What was different from these findings in our study, the patients with CRPS continued to lose their hand bone mineral density on the fracture side during one year unlike the patient group without CRPS. This interesting finding suggested that other than the effect of immobilisation itself, some of the clinical parameters particularly CRPS might be effective in progressive hand bone loss which was detectable by hand DEXA.

Similar to our results, in a prospective study investigating the effect of CRPS on osteoporosis after tibial fractures in 60 patients, it has been reported that patients with CRPS lost significantly more bone mineral than those without during one year (2). Region-specific osteoporosis which is characterized by elevated bone turnover and bone resorption was accepted as one of the comorbidities of CPRS (6,24) The well-known periarticular patchy osteoporosis, which can be seen on X-ray pictures and so-called high-turnover osteoporosis with increased osteo-clastic activity by neural inflammatory factors, especially TNF-alpha and Substance P (24). This clinical condition is important because it has been re-ported that CRPS was associated with a rare complication, occurring in less than 2 % of fractures, especially in lower extremity after minimal trauma (1,8). In a case report of a competitive athlete having CRPS in one extremity after overex-ertion, it has been shown that his bone density was low in affected lower extremity and normal at non-CRPS sites, potentially exposing him to greater risk of fra-gility fracture in the affected regions (8). Likewise in these studies, the continua-tion of hand bone loss during one year in patients with CRPS unlike the patients without showed us that CRPS was very important factor for regional osteopo-rosis. It might be due to neural inflammation pathogenesis or upper limb dys-function depending on the symptoms of CRPS. Despite its importance, the number of studies were very limited in the literature. Additionally, all of these studies were related with lower extremity fractures in the literature. Our study was the first one investigating the effect of CRPS on regional osteoporosis by hand DEXA after DRF. This is one of the major strength of our study. Regarding clinical parameters, our results showed that parameters related with pain and upper limb dysfunction were more severely affected in patients with CRPS when compared to those of without CRPS. Studies demonstrated that the normal course of recovery following a distal radius fracture is one where severe symptoms subside within the first two months (25). However, this is not the case for CRPS. Although properly treated, patients with CRPS of upper limb may continue to have sequel signs and symptoms of the disease in long term (8–60 months) (26) This is not surprising because it has been known that CRPS is a complex disorder resulting in chronic pain and kinesiophobia and therefore difficulty in rehabili-tation further and disability and fracture (6).Similarly in our study, patients with CRPS showed some improvement in clinical parameters but couldn't decrease as much as to the level of those without CRPS. They had still residual symptoms after one year. This picture as a whole affects the health-related quality of life and places a huge emotional and psychological burden on patients (6). Therefore clinicians should pay attention to this complex disorder in order to prevent fur-ther complications and disability. Another interesting finding of this study is that, there was a negative relationship with the bone loss and severity of CRPS (evaluated by SHSS), pain severity (according to VAS), and dysfunction of the upper limb (by DASH) in patients with CRPS. As the scores of clinical parameters increase, the amount of hand bone loss decrease. Hovever, these scores were not correlated with hand BMD in patients without CRPS. These results showed us that the severity of CPRS together with pain and upper limb dysfunction might be important factor on hand bone loss other than the effect of immobilization itself. In our study, the severity of CRPS was detected by SHSS and this scoring system has been used to evaluate the severity of the symptoms of CRPS (16) The higher the scores, the more severe the CRPS, and this severity was found to be correlated with the loss of hand BMD. This is not surprising because its under-lying mechanism is somewhat different. Since it is becoming to be accepted as a novel autoinflammatory disease, the whole clinical spectrum is related to neural inflammatory factors (calcitonin gene-related peptide, substance P, TNF-alpha, and NGF) (24). All clinical signs of CRPS including osteoporosis have been linked to neurogenic inflammatory peptides (24). The more severe the neural inflammation, the more severe the pain, dysfunction, and osteoporosis. Depending on the severity of underlying neural inflammation, clinical patterns might be variable (26). It might spread ipsilaterally to the proximal of the extremity and even to the contralateral extremity (26,27). Therefore CRPS results in severe upper extremity dysfunction from distal to proximal and causes inability to participate in daily activities and eventually aggravating the osteopo-rosis (2,8). It has been reported that in those patients in whom severe symptoms of CRPS have severe extremity dysfunction the use of extremity reduces in long-term (4). This may result in delay in return to work and has long-term social and economic implications (4). Savas et al. (26) investigated the effect of symptoms of CRPS on function and daily activities, and they found functional impairment in patients with CRPS was maintained and it could be detected on the basis of DASH(28). Additionally, DASH has been reported to address global upper-extremity disability and symptoms, including physical, social, and psychological items and also found to be sensitive to clinical changes in patients with DRF (29). In our study we have evaluated the upper extremity dysfunction by DASH. Supporting the findings in the literature, our results showed that total scores were significantly higher in patients with CRPS than those of without. Additionally, the more severe the dysfunction scores, the more severe the hand bone loss at the end of one year. Our study is the first one showing this relation-ship that is another strength. Therefore it might be suggested that, clinicians should be aware of the patients having CRPS at the initial phase of the treatment and follow-up these patients carefully. Because they might be under risk of further fracture during rehabilitation, special exercises should be programmed according to these individuals.

Conclusion

As a conclusion, we recommend the incorporation of DXA measurements in the clinical care of patients with CRPS after DRF. Because it is not only accurate and also feasible requiring minimal patient preparation and time consuming. By means of hand DEXA, it might be possible to eliminate the risky patients having regional osteoporosis for further fracture and disability. This is crucially important factor during rehabilitation process for the rehabilitation team. According to results of our study bone loss after distal forearm fracture continued to decrease after one year significantly. And this loss was found to be related to severity of CRPS, pain, and upper limb dysfunction. That means, patients especially having higher scores symptoms of CRPS and upper limb dysfunction according to clinical measures (with DASH and SHSS) had further hand bone loss during one year. Therefore, it should be kept in mind that bone loss might be continued over one year after fracture, and strategies improving bone strength, including both pharmacological and non-pharmacological initiatives should be designed accordingly. Rehabilitation strategies should be oriented to improve upper limb function. Although our results are promising about this issue, further studies are needed to confirm our results.

Limitations of the Research

There are some limitations. These are sample size, insurance coverage of DEXA scans (covered by public insurance), lack of some objective clinical tests such as bone resorption biomarkers, electrophysiological, and autonomical tests etc. Further studies are still needed including larger sample size and considering objective clinical tests.

Author Contributions

Concept – J:Ö.; Design – J.Ö:A.Ü.; Analysis and/or Interpretation -.JÖ.,BK,KA; Literature Review – J.Ö., BK,KA. Writing Manuscript – J.Ö.K.A .; Critical Review – BK,JÖ.

Conflict of İnterest

There is no conflict of interest by the authors.

Financial Disclosure

The authors declared that they did not receive financial support for this study.

References

1. Alenfeld,F.E., Diessel,E. & Brezger,M. et al. (2000). Detailed Analyses in Periarticular Osteoporosis in Rheumatoid Arthritis. Osteoporos Int., 11: 400–7.

2. Alexandre,C. & Vico, L. (2011). Pathophysiology of Bone Loss in Disuse Osteoporosis. *Joint Bone Spine*. Dec; 78(6): 572–6.

3. Beleckas, C., Calfee, R. (2017). Distal radius fractures in the Athlete. *Curr Rev Musculoskelet Med.*, Mar; 10(1): 62–71.

4. Birklein, F., Schmelz, M.(2008). Neuropeptides, Neurogenic Inflammation and Complex Regional Pain Syndrome (CRPS). *Neuroscience Letters*, 437: 199–202

5. Carlsson M.A. (1983). Assessment of Chronic Pain. Aspects of the Reliability and Validity of the Visual Analogue Scale. *Pain*, 16: 87–101

6. Deodha, R.A., Brabyn, J., Jones, P.W., Davis, M. J. & Woolf, A.D.(1995). Longitudinal Study of Hand Bone Densitometry in Rheumatoidarthritis. *ArthrandRheum*, 38(9): 1204–1210.

7. Dilek, B., Ayhan, Ç., Yagci, G. & Yakut, Y.2018). Effectiveness of the Graded Motor Imagery to Improve Hand Function in Patients with Distal Radius Fracture: A Randomized Controlled Trial. J Hand Ther. 2018 Jan - Mar;31(1):2-9.e1

8. Eyres, K.S., Kanis, J.A. (1995). Bone Loss after Tibial Fracture. *J Bone JointSurg., [Br]*:77-B: 473–8.

9. Feng, X., Mc Donald, J.M. (2011). Disorders of Bone Remodelling. *Annu Rev Pathol.*, 6: 121–145.

10. Goh, E.L. & Chidambaram, S.Ma.D. (2017). Complex Regional Pain Syndrome: A Recent update. *Burns Trauma.*, 5: 2.3-5

11. Harden, N.R., Bruehl, S., Perez, S.G.M., Birklein, F., Marinus, J., Maihofner, C., et al. (2010). Validation of Proposed Diagnostic Criteria (the "Budapest Criteria") for Complex Regional Pain Syndrome. *Pain*. 150(2): 268–274,

12. Hartwig, M., Gelbrich, G., Griewing, B. (2012). Functional Orthosis in Shoulder Joint Subluxation after Ischaemic Brain Stroke to Avoid Posthemiplegic Shoulder-Hand Syndrome: Randomized cCinical tTial. *Clin Rehabil.*, 26: 807–816.

13. Haugeberg, G., Green, M.J. & Conaghan, P.G., et al. (2007). Hand Bone Densitometry: A Moresensitive Standard for the Assessment of Early Bone Damage in Rheumatoid Arthritis. *Ann Rheum Dis.*, 66: 1513–1517.

14. Hind, K., Johnson, M. (2014). Complex Regional Pain Syndrome in a Competitive Athlete and Regional Osteoporosis Assessed by Dual-Energy X-ray Absorptiometry: A Case Report. *Journal of Medic Case Reports.*, 8: 165.2-4

15. Hoff, M., Kvien, T.K., Kalvesten, J., Elden, A. & Haugeberg, G. (2009). Adalimumab Therapy Reduces Hand Bone Loss in Early Rheumatoid Arthritis: Explorative Analyses from the PREMIER Study. *Ann Rheum Dis.*, 68: 1171–1176.

16. Ingle, B.M., Hay, S.M., Bottjer, H.M., et al. (1999). Chances in Bone Mass and Bone Turnover Following Distal Forearm Fracture. *Osteoporosis International*, 10: 399–407.

17. Karacan, I., Aydin, T., Ozaras, N. (2004). Thirty-Two Patients with CRPS-1 of the Hand: Bone Loss in the Contralateral Asymptomatic Hand in Patients with Complex Regional Pain Syndrometype-I. *J Bone Miner Metab.*, 22(1): 44–7.

18. Kendall, F.P., McCreary, E.K., & Provance, P.G. (1993). Joint Motions. In: Butler JP, (Ed). *Muscles Testing and Function*. Baltimore, MD: Williams and Wilkins.

19. Kessous, R., Weintraub, A.Y., Mattan, Y., Dresner-Pollak, R., Brezis, M., Liebergall, M., Kandel, L.(2014). Improving Compliance to Osteoporosis Work Up and Treatment in Postmenopausal Patients after a Distal Radius Fracture. *Taiwanese Journal of Obstetrics & Gynecology.*, 53: 206–209.

20. Kumar, V., Kalita, J., Gujral, R.B. et al. (2 001): A Study of Bone Densitometry in Patients with Complex Regional Pain Syndrome after Stroke. *Postgrad Med J.*, 77: 519–522.

21. Lau, R.Y., Guo, X.(2011). Review on Current Osteoporosis Research: With Special Focus on Disuse Bone Loss. *J Osteoporosis.*, 293808:1–6.:.

22. MacDermid, J.C., Roth, J.H., Richards, R.S. (2003). Pain and Disability Reported in the Year Following a Distal Radius Fracture: A Cohort Study. *BMC Musculoskelet Disord.*; 4:24.

23. Mathiowetz, V., Weber, K., Volland, G., et al. (1984). Reliability and Validity of Grip and Pinch Strenghth Evaluations. *J Hand Surg.*, 9: 222–226.

24. Sarangi, P.P., Ward, A.J. & Atkins, R.M. (1992). Fractures after Regional Disuse Osteoporosis: Case Report. *J OrthopRheum.*, 5: 233–7.

25. Saranghi, P.P., Ward, A.J., Smith, E.J. & Staddon, G.E. (1993). Atkins RM. Algodistrophy and Osteoporosis after Tibial Fractures. *J Bone JointSurg [Br]*:75-B: 450–2.

26. Savas,S., Baloğlu, H.H. & Ay, G.(2009). The Effect of Sequel Symptoms and Signs of Complex Regional Pain Syndrome Type 1 on Upper Extremity Disability and Quality of lLfe. *Rheum Int.*, 29: 545-547.

27. Schmidt, R.T. & Toews, J.V.(1970). Grip Strength as Measured by the Jamar Dynamometer. *Arch Phys Med Rehabil.*, 51: 321–327.

28. Smet, L.D., SooHoo, N.F. & McDonald, A.P.et al. (2008). The DASH Questionnaire and Score in the Evaluation of Hand and Wrist Disorders. *Acta Orthop. Belg.*, 74: 575–581

29. Van, R.,A., Marinus, J., Putter, H., Sarah, R., Bosselaar, J., Lorimer, G. et al. (2011). Spreading of Complex Regional Pain Syndrome Not a Random Process. *J NeuralTransm.*, Sep; 118(9): 1301–1309.

Emel Özcan, Kerem Alptekin, Bilal Uysal, Bahar Teksöz, Halim İşsever, and E. Ece Özcan Ekşi

The Prevalance of Musculoskeletal Diseases and the Physical Risk Factors in Metal Workers

Abstract: *Introduction:* Metal workers are under the risk of musculoskeletal disorders because of great physical efforts are required.

Objective: To determine the prevalence and physical risk factors of MSD among metal workers.

Methods: The study has been done in metal industry factories at Istanbul and nearby. 1000 questionnaires sent, only 130 of them returned. The questionnaire included personal characteristics and working conditions. Test-Re-test reliability study of questionnaire was performed. Pearson, Chi Square vs Fisher's Exact Test were used for statistical analysis.

Results: Prevalence of MSD in last 12 months was 83,07 %. The most frequent three areas of pain were low back with 64.8%, back with 52,9% neck with 48%.

Most significant relations were as at the below when work activities were separately assessed as risk factors; back pain among people, lifting 20 kg frequently at work was 52,6 % (p=0.003), shoulder pain among people pulling 20 kg load was 80 %(p= 0.001), elbow pain among people carrying 20 kg was 72.2 %(p = 0.001), back pain among people working with reaching hands and arms more than 2 hours was 73 %(p =0.000), low back pain among people standing on their feet frequently more than 2 hours was 72.2 % (p=0.008). Sixty-seven of workers (51,5 %) applied to physician because of complaints and 42 of workers (33.1 %) received reports and were absent from work because of MSD.

Conclusion: We suppose that participatory ergonomics program can prevent metal workers from MSD.

Keywords: Musculoskeletal Disorders, Metal Workers, Risk Factors, Ergonomics

Introduction

Work-related musculoskeletal diseases (WRMSD), which develop as a result of work-related activities, are a common health problem in developed and developing countries, and those are the leading causes of disability. WRMSD affects muscles, tendons, ligaments, nerves, and other support structures of the body. First, it affects the low back, neck, hands, wrists, elbows, and shoulders. WRMSD symptoms are pain, discomfort, fatigue, numbness, tingling, movement restriction, and disability (1).

The role of some physical and psychosocial factors such as weight lifting, transportation, rotation activities in the workplace causes WRMSD and that has been proven in past studies. WRMSD is evaluated with the use of self-reported questionnaires in the studies. WRMSD affects employees, employers, insurance systems, and the country's economy, with a high cost to society due to high working day loss and insurance compensation payments. In the United States, the National Academy of Sciences reports that the total expenditure incurred in 2005 for MKİH exceeded US $ 1 trillion. (2)

In almost every workplace and occupational group there is a risk for WRMSD. Metal work is considered to be a hard and intensive work that requires high physical and aerobic loading. In the UK, Europe, and South-East Asia, metal workers are reported to be at high risk for musculoskeletal disorders, especially in the low back, neck, shoulders, wrists, and hands.

Materials and Methods

Objective

To determine the prevalence and physical risk factors of MSD among metal workers.

The Universe and Sample of Research

The study was carried out in the metal industry factories where the members of the United Metal Workers Union worked in Istanbul and its surrounding provinces. 130 metal workers, adults, male participants voluntarily participated the study (n=130).

Data Collection Tools and Data Collection

Research Data

A questionnaire was applied to 130 people working in metal works. The questionnaire included personal characteristics, work, and work characteristics. Musculoskeletal complaints were questioned by Nordic Musculoskeletal Questionnaire. A more detailed back pain questionnaire was applied to participants who have low back pain.

Data Analysis

The pre-test of the questionnaire was performed for the test-retest reliability. Pearson, Chi Square and Fisher's Exact Test were used for statistical analysis.

Ethical Aspects of Research

Permission was obtained from the Istanbul University Ethics Board for Clinical Research and the United Metal Workers Union for research.

Result

All of the 130 participants were male (100 %). The prevalence of musculoskeletal disorders in the last 12 months was 83.07 %. 95 of 130 participants (73 %) worked in the automotive sector and 35 of 130 participants (27 %) in the casting sector (Fig 1). The mean age was 34 (18–53) years. There was no statistically significant difference between the two sectors and the complaints distribution.

Neck, back, and low back pain were most common in the thirties ages. When the prevalence of pain complaints in the last 12 months were investigated according to regions, it was on the waist 64.8 %, back 52.9 %, neck 48.0 %, shoulder 41.3 %, knees 36.3 %, hands 31.1 %, foot 30.6 %, and hips 29.3 % (Fig. 2).

The prevalence of musculoskeletal complaints was 66 % in the last week. When the criterion of adherence to the job was investigated, this criterion was determined in 89.23 %. The most significant relationship was established between back pain and work adherence (p = 0.000, p <0.05). When the prevalence of pain complaints in the last week were investigated according to the regions, it was on the waist 51.6 %, back 35.8 %, neck 31.5 %, shoulder 32.1 %, knees 25.2 %, hands 22.6 %, feet 22.5 %, and hips 20.1 % (Fig. 3).

When the risk factors are evaluated, there was a statistically significant relationship between 20 kg load lifting and shoulder, back, and lumbar pain; 20 kg

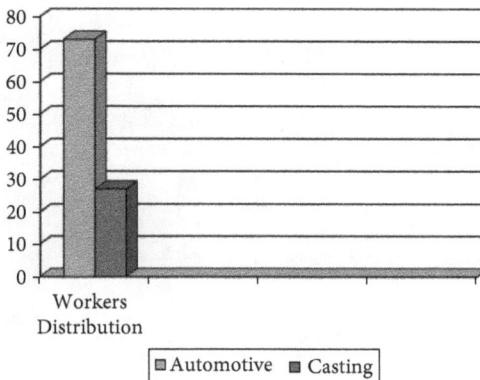

Fig. 1: Sectoral Distribution of Workers in the Study

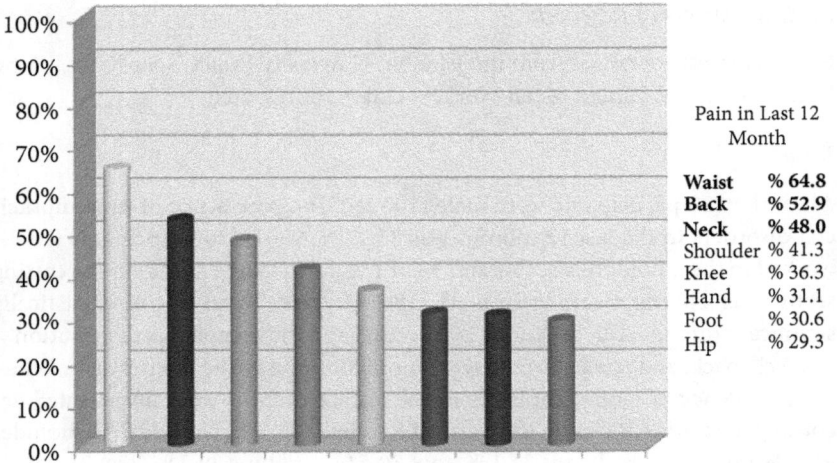

Pain in Last 12
Month

Waist	**% 64.8**
Back	**% 52.9**
Neck	**% 48.0**
Shoulder	% 41.3
Knee	% 36.3
Hand	% 31.1
Foot	% 30.6
Hip	% 29.3

Fig. 2: Regional Distribution of Pain in the Last 12 Months

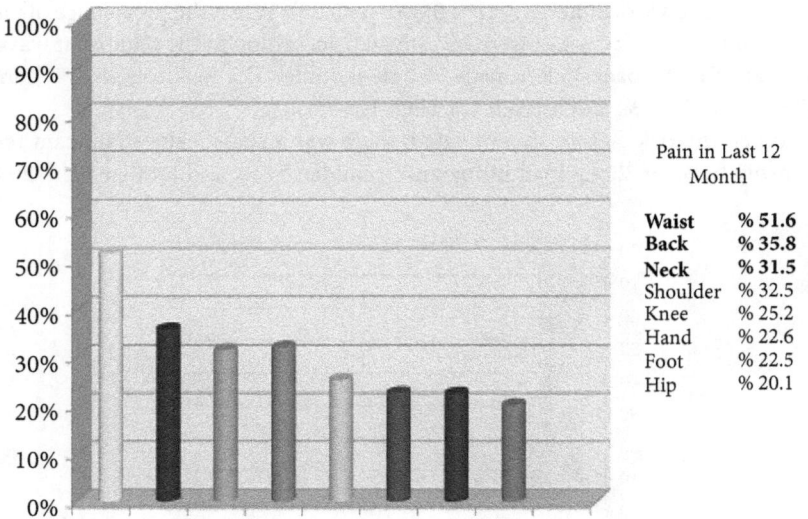

Pain in Last 12
Month

Waist	**% 51.6**
Back	**% 35.8**
Neck	**% 31.5**
Shoulder	% 32.5
Knee	% 25.2
Hand	% 22.6
Foot	% 22.5
Hip	% 20.1

Fig. 3: Regional Distribution of Pain in the Last Week

Tab. 1: Relationship Between Lifting, Pulling, Carrying of the 20 Kg Load and Pain

	20kg Load Lifting	20kg Load Pulling	20kg Load Carrying
Back Pain	% 52,6	% 74.1	% 50,9
Shoulder Pain	% 54,5	% 80	% 53,7
Low Back Pain	% 48,5	% 70	% 48,5

load pull and the neck, back, waist, hip, knee, and hand pain; and 20 kg load carrying the weight, neck, shoulder, waist, back, and elbow pain.

When the work-related activities were evaluated separately as risk factors, the most significant relationships were as follows: workers frequently working with 20 kg load lifting had back pain was 52.6 % (p=0.003, p <0.05), workers frequently working with 20 kg load pull had shoulder pain was 80 % (p= 0.001, p <0.05), workers frequently working with 20 kg load carrying had elbow pain was 72.2% (p = 0.001, p <0.05), workers frequently working with position of arms and hands extended had back pain 73 % (p =0.000, p <0.05), and workers frequently standing and working for more than two hours had waist pain 72.2 % (p = 0.008, p <0.05).

Non-work-related diseases were detected as follows: 3 patients had diabetes, 2 had inflammatory rheumatism, 2 had thyroid disease, and 2 had psychological disorders. Sixty five (51.5 %) of the employees applied to the doctor about musculoskeletal disorders; 42 employees (33.1 %) reported that they used reports due to musculoskeletal disorders and could not go to work.

Conclusion

People who work with metals, requiring heavy physical activity, are at high risk for musculoskeletal diseases. According to Burdof et al., 283 male metal workers were followed for 2 years due to musculoskeletal diseases. In 12-month follow-up, workers had pain at low back 41 %, neck 20 %, back 22 %, foot and ankle 33 %, and 51 % of employees could not continue to work due to musculoskeletal discomfort. (3)

In the cross-sectional study by Hussain et al., 461 trucks construction workers were surveyed by Nordic Questionnaire. Musculoskeletal discomfort in the last year was detected 79 %. The most common effected sites were the low back 65 %, the back 60 %, and the shoulders 57 % (4).

According to Gangopadhyay et al. the prevalence of upper extremity musculoskeletal diseases among rice workers in India, the most common effected sites, was determined as hands, wrists, fingers, and shoulders. It was determined that dealing with repetitive jobs and hammering caused wrist and shoulder pain.(5)

Poosanthanasarn et al. examined the health status of workers in automobile industry in Eastern Thailand; 172 workers were evaluated; the incidence of occupational accidents was higher in patients with muscle pain. Small and large pressing machines were found to be effective in the development of musculoskeletal disorders. (6)

In the study which evaluated the frequency of musculoskeletal disorders in unionized iron workers in the UK declared that the areas of disorders were detected: low back 56 %, wrist and fingers 40 %, and pain frequency detected 36 %. The most frequently diagnosed disorders by the workplace physician were Tendinitis (19 %), ruptured disc (18 %), bursitis in the shoulder (15 %), and Carpal Tunnel Syndrome (12 %) (7).

Wang et al. musculoskeletal disorders in metal workers in the USA in 1992–2014 were examined and 40 % of the patients had low back pain. In our study, the prevalence of lower back pain was 64.8 %. Another noteworthy factor in the United States is the doubling of the numbers of the group between the 55–64 ages, between 1992 and 2014 years. In our study, the mean age was 34 (18–53) years. This situation can be explained by the fact that in developed countries such as the USA, heavy and dangerous businesses are now less preferred (8).

We didn't examine environmental factors in detail such as humidity or pollution of the air. Saha et al. found a high rate of fluoride in their urine, and found a statistically significant relationship between these conditions and musculoskeletal diseases (OR: 2.71; 95 % CI: 1.81–3.75).

In our study we didn't apply any ergonomic intervention or treatment. There are not many studies in the literature.(9,10) According to Burger et al., 38 metal workers were divided into two groups. One group received a stochastic resonance total body vibration device at a frequency ranging from 1 to 12 Hz for 3 minutes over a period of 4 minutes, while the other group was not treated. In the next 4 weeks the groups were replaced. At the end of the study, musculoskeletal pain was significantly decreased in the treated group compared to the other group (p <0.01).

Also it has been the subject of research which specific tasks of metal workers increase the musculoskeletal complaints. In our study, 20 kg load is a threshold value for the emergence of disorders. In particular, the 20 kg load pulling realized with non-ergonomic posture may lead to the highest rate of pain in the back, waist, and shoulder area. Choi et al. using a body map, identified green, yellow, and red colors as the most painful area of the person. Besides, it was observed that the rebar clamping movement caused the highest hand clamping power with dynamometer (11).

Results

In our study, the prevalence of musculoskeletal disorders in metal workers was similar with other countries. Weight lifting and the use of inappropriate body mechanics were determined as risk factors.

As a result, metal workers who require heavy physical activity are at high risk for musculoskeletal disorders. In order to take these risks under control, participatory ergonomics programs, ergonomics trainings, and ergonomics arrangements in the workplace should be established and their effectiveness should be investigated.

Limitations of the Research

One of the limitations of our study is the lack of any intervention related to treatment. On the other hand we did not investigate the working environment properly. So we might have missed some environmental factors, causing diseases as well.

Author Contributions

Concept - EÖ.; Design – E.Ö., H.K.A.; Analysis and/or Interpretation – H.İ .; Literature Review – B.U.,E.E.Ö Writing Manuscript – H.K.A, B.T .; Critical Review – E.Ö., H.K.A.

Conflict of Interest

There is no conflict of interest by the authors.

Financial Disclosure

The authors declared that they did not receive financial support for this study.

References

1. Amell, T., Kumar, S. (2002). Work-Related Musculoskeletal Disorders: Design as a Preventive Strategy. A Review, *Jornual of Occupational Rehabilitation*. 4: 255–264.
2. Burdorf,A.,Naaktgeboren,B.&Post,W.(1998). Prognostic Factors for Musculoskeletal Sickness Absence and Return to Work among Welders and Metal Workers. *Occup Environ Med*. 55: 490– 495

3. Burger, C., Schade, V., Lindner, C., Radlinger, L. & Elfering, A. (2012). Stochastic Resonance Training Reduces Musculoskeletal Symptoms in Metal Manufacturing Workers: A Controlled Preventive Intervention Study. *Work*. 42(2): 269–278.

4. Choi, S.D. (2010). Ergonomic Assessment of Musculoskeletal Discomfort of Iron Workers in Highway Construction. *Work*. 36(1): 47–53.

5. Gangopadhyay,S.,Ghosh,T.,Das,T.,Ghosahal,G.&DasB.B. (2007). Prevelance of Upper Limb Musculoskeletal Disorders among Brass Metal Workers in West Bengal. *Industrial Health*. India. 45: 365–370.

6. Martin, S.F.,Laura, P.& David, H. (2005). Prevalence of Musculoskeletal Disorders in Union Ironworkers. *Journal of Occupational and Environmental Hygiene* 2: 4,203–212.

7. Melhorn, J.M., Gardner, P., (2004). How We Prevent Prevention of Musculoskeletal Disordes in the Workplace. Clin Orthop. 419: 285–296.

8. Poosanthanasarn,N.&Lohachit,C.(2005). The Health of Workers in a Metal Autoparts Factory in Eastern Thailand, *Southeast Asian J Trop Med Public Health*. 36(3): 783–789.

9. Tokeer,H. (2004) Musculoskeletal Symptoms among Truck Assembly Workers. *Occupational Medicine*, 54: 506–512

10. Saha,A.,Mukherjee,A.K.&Ravichandran,B.(2016). Musculoskeletal Problems and Fluoride Exposure: A Cross-Sectional Study among Metal Smelting Workers. *Toxicol Ind Health*, 32(9):1581–1588.

11. Wang,X.,Dong,X.S.,Choi,S.D.&Dement,J.(2017). Work-Related Musculoskeletal Disorders among Construction Workers in the United States from 1992 to 2014. *Occup Environ Med*. 74(5): 374–380.

Ömer Şevgin, Kerem Alptekin, Bülent Aksoy, and Jülide Öncü Alptekin

Evaluation of the Effectiveness of Home Exercise Program Method with Attention Level and Tampa Kinesiophobia Scale

Abstract: Objective: With that study we aimed to compare home exercises and video-based exercises regarding attention level and kinesiophobia.

Material and Methods: The patients over 65 years who are living in Beşiktaş, district of İstanbul and who have physical therapy services in Beşiktaş. Sixteen participants were randomly assigned to 2 groups. The first group was recommended for home exercises by physiotherapist in line with the treatments video; the second group was recommended by the publication. Then, the Number Range Test (WMS-2) and the Mental Coordination Test (WMS-3) were used to evaluate the levels of caution in the patients in each of the two groups. Pain and movement fear evaluations were repeated after 15 days of exercise program. In addition, patients' quality of life was also evaluated. Pain scores of the patients were measured before and after treatment with Visual Analog Scala (VAS); Exercise avoidance (fear) scores with the Tampa Kinesiophobia Scale; the quality of life was measured with short form (SF-36). The 15-day exercise frequency between the groups and its relationship with other parameters were compared.

Results: The research was a cohort study and parametric tests were used and analyzed by normalization. The patients' disease and education levels were heterogeneous and differences were present. Video exercises increased the frequency of exercise more than exercises prescribed on paper.

Discussion: Low number of patients, heterogeneous patient population and lack of pain constitute the weaknesses of our study. In exercise applications, cognitive levels of elderly patients may affect the correct and complete exercise.

Conclusions: Patients' pain and fear of movement are reduced by exercise. However, the video exercises were superior than exercises prescribed on paper. In our study, the relationship between the patient's attention level and the frequency of exercise were also investigated.

Keywords: Physiotherapy, Exercise therapy, Quality of life, Video-based exercises

Introduction

Exercise; it is a subset of physical activity, expressed as planned, structured, and repetitive movement. It is aimed to develop and protect one or more components of physical fitness. Only 28 % of the population over 12 years of age in Turkey is to make exercise on a regular basis.(1) In addition, as the age progresses, the rate of those who do not exercise at all increases up to 80 %. Matthieu Boisgontier et al. in his research: A group of young adults seated in front of the computer was commanded by the symbolic screen character, and the subjects were shown small images that then appeared and disappeared, describing physical activity or inactivity. It was found that subjects who needed to act quickly to the physical activity image were generally successful. However, during the movement, the activity of the brain waves was found to work more in order to avoid the image of brain inactivity. (2) It is seen that the results give the idea that immobility is attractive to our brain from creation. In the study conducted by Nicolson et al. 341 patients over age 50 were divided into 3 groups by stopping exercise. In the rapid decrease in adherence to exercise group, in the 12-week numerical ranking scale, from 7.7 ± 1.6; 4.2 ± 2.2 was regressed within 22 weeks. In the moderately decreasing group, this ratio decreased from 8.5 ± 1.5 to 7.8 ± 1.5.(3) This study emphasizes the high dropout rates in home exercise programs and the need to closely monitor patients. The way the exercises are administered affects the treatment process at different levels. Exercise at home or clinic, or self-application of exercise by the patient or under the supervision of a physiotherapist leads to different results.

While some studies show that the home exercises are more effective, some studies show that hospitalized exercises are more effective.(4,5) Tunay et al. divided 60 patients with knee osteoarthritis into two groups. One group was given home exercise and the other group was given exercise in the hospital under the supervision of physiotherapist. As a result of the study, there was a significant improvement in VAS and Timed Up and Go test in the hospital-based exercise group compared to the home exercise group.(6) There are several studies showing that the way home exercises are given to patients affect the quality of treatment. Supporting home exercise programs with written and visual materials positively affects the effectiveness of the treatment. For example, in COPD patients, within the virtual reality application with the help of a three-dimensional sensor, the exercises are made fun and the effectiveness of the treatment is increased. (7)

In a systematic review Axel Georg et al, in this study, the effectiveness of Electronic Health-supported home exercise programs, which are different for the patients with knee osteoarthritis, and in general, e-health-supported exercise interventions, small short- and long-term positive effects on pain, physical function, and QL in OAC patients have been emphasized. (8) For the purpose of the study, the effects of home exercise programs on the pain level and movement fear of the patients were examined and the effect of home exercise programs on the frequency of exercise was compared with the frequency of exercise.

Materials and Methods

The sample of the study consisted of 32 patients residing in Beşiktaş, Istanbul and receiving physical therapy and rehabilitation services at home. To work; Patients aged 65 years and over, patients who were recommended to exercise, and patients who read the information form and signed the consent form were included. Exclusion criteria are; Patients under 65 years of age are those who have not read the consent form and have not signed the consent form and have uncontrolled systemic disease. The patients in the research sample were given the exercises in their own homes. Participants, who were randomly assigned to two equal groups of 16, were subjected to the Number Range Test (WMS-2) and Mental Coordination Test (WMS-3). Measurement results were used to create subgroups.(9,10)

Data Collection Tools and Data Collection

In each group, the average of the test results was obtained and the level of attention was higher than 8 people who were above the average; The remaining 8 people were classified as low level of attention. After the subgroups of the sample are created, respectively, pain assessment with VAS and fear of motion with a Tampa Kinesiophobia scale were evaluated.(11) The exercise follow-up form was then delivered to the patient for daily filling. Exercise follow-up form is a stylish form of 'yes' and 'no' in the history of the day. When the patient did the exercise on a daily basis, he was asked to mark 'no' when he didn't. First group exercises were given by video; the second group was given with the letter. At the end of the exercise program, VAS and taping kinesiophobia and SF-36 (quality of life) tests were performed.(12) Exercise follow-up form was delivered to the patient on the first day. First and last tests were compared and evaluated with frequency of exercise.

Evaluation tests of the study were parametric tests and normality analyzes were performed. Demographic *data of the patients included in the study were requested and recorded* (Tab. 1).

Ethical Aspects of Research

Ethics committee approval was obtained from Bahçeşehir University Clinical Research Ethics Commission. Municipality health directorate was contacted and

Tab. 1: Demographic Data of the Patients

		Video		Written	
		n	Percent	n	Percent
Gender	Male	6	60,0	4	40,0
	Female	10	45,5	12	54,5
Education	Primary school	4	40,0	6	60,0
	Middle school	2	40,0	3	60,0
	High school	7	66,7	4	33,3
	University	3	50,0	3	50,0
Main Complaint	Leg pain	0	0	1	100,0
	Back pain	3	100,0	0	0,0
	Disc herniation	2	33,3	4	66,7
	Knee pain	1	100,0	0	0
	Knee prsothesis	1	50,0	1	50,0
	Femur fracture	2	50,0	2	50,0
	Fibromyalgia	1	100,0	0	0,0
	Hemiplegia	0	0,0	1	100,0
	Coxartrosis	1	100,0	0	0,0
	Meniscectomy	1	100,0	0	0,0
	Shoulder pain	2	66,7	1	33,3
	Osteoarthritis	2	66,7	1	33,3
	Parkinson	0	0,0	2	100,0
	Skoliosis	0	0,0	1	100,0
	Spinal stenosis	0	0,0	2	100,0
WMS Grade	Low attention	2	20,0	8	80,0
	High attention	14	63,6	8	36,4
Target Grade	Low attention	6	37,5	10	62,5
	High attention	10	62,5	6	37,5
SF Grading	Low Life Quality	6	37,5	10	62,5
	High Life Quality	10	62,5	6	37,5

information about the study was given and written permission was obtained. Participants received written and verbal consent to participate in the study.

Discussion

Patients with different diseases were included in the study; however, there is no classification according to the diseases. A heterogeneous group was included

Tab. 2: Comparison of VAS Values

Video	N	Mean	Std. Deviation	t	P
VAS 1	16	6,96	1,01	9,037	0,000
VAS 2	16	2,81	1,52		
Written	**N**	**Mean**	**Std. Deviation**	**t**	**P**
VAS 1	16	6,26	1,37	7,854	0,000
VAS 2	16	3,38	1,63		

VAS 1 mean value was 6.96 in the video group, while the mean VAS 2 value was 2.81. The mean VAS 2 was significantly lower than the VAS 1 mean. (P <0.05) The mean value of VAS 1 was 6.26 in the group, while the average of the VAS 2 measurements was 3.38 (Table 2). It was also found meaningful. According to the results of t-test in the independent groups in the video and group, the mean of the frequency of exercise according to the WMS classes and the difference between these averages are significant; while the average of people with low levels of attention in the group is 22; the average of people with high levels of attention to exercise was 22.66.

Tab. 3: Attention Level of Patients

Video Group WMS grading		N	Mean	Std. Deviation	t	P
Exercise Frequency	Low attention	2	22,00	1,41	-0,150	0,883
	High attention	14	22,66	5,99		
Written Group WMS grading						
ExExercise	Low attention	8	15,50	3,74	-1,832	0,088
Frequency	High attention	8	20,11	6,06		

There was no significant difference between two groups according to t-test results. On the other hand, in the video group, the average exercise level of people with low attention level was 15,50; the average of people with high attention level was 20,11. No significant difference was found in this group (Table 3)

in the study because of the wide range of diseases in the sample of the study. Therefore, we do not mention any finding of our study on the effectiveness of home exercise according to the type of disease. In addition, it is thought that cognitive levels of elderly patients may affect the application of exercises in video and fiction. In our study, it is not possible to make an evaluation about the findings in the literature since no measurement was made about the exercise types other than home exercise.

Tab. 4: Frequency of Exercises

Group		N	Mean	Std. Deviation	t	P
Exercise Frequency	Video	16	22,58	5,59	2,450	0,020
	Written	16	17,81	5,42		

According to the results of t-test in independent groups for the comparison of the frequency of exercise in video and group groups; while the average frequency of exercise in the video group was 22.58; The average frequency of exercise was 17,81. According to t-test results in independent groups; there was a significant difference between the mean frequency of video and group exercises (p <0.05) (Table 4).

Tab. 5: Tampa Kinesiophobia Measurements

		N	Mean	Std. Deviation	t	P
Video Group	TK First	16	47,75	4,71	2,213	0,043
	TK Last	16	45,75	2,74		
Written Group	TK First	16	48,69	4,22	1,202	0,248
	TK Last	16	47,69	5,28		

According to the results of the t-test, the first and the last measurements of the Tampa Kinesiophobia scale in the video group were compared. Tampa Kinesiophobia first measurement was 47.75; the second measurement average was 45.75. According to the results of t-test in the dependent groups, it was significantly different between the first and the last measurement (p <0.05). In the written exercise group, the mean of Tampa Kinesiophobia was 48.69 and the second was 47.69, and there was no significant difference between the first and the last measurements (Table 5).

Tab. 6: Correlation of Exercise Frequency and SF-36

Video Group		Exercise Frequency	SF-36 Score	Written Group		Exercise Frequency	SF-36 Score
Exercise	R	1	-,325	Exercise	R	1	,400
Frequency	P		,219	Frequency	P		,125
SF-36 Score	R	-,325	1	VAS Change	R	,400	1
	P	,219			P	,125	

Correlation analysis was performed to determine the relationship between SF-36 score and frequency of exercise in the video and group, and Pearson correlation coefficient was obtained. There was no significant relationship between SF-36 score and frequency of exercise in video and group (p> 0.05) (Table 6).

Conclusion

With the development of technology, new methods are emerging in the ways in which hospitals are given both in hospitals and at home.(13) The exercise with video is also one of themIn our study, it was investigated whether the exercises given with video were superior to the exercises given by the manuscript. In addition, the effect of patients' attention level on treatment was also investigated. According to the findings of our research, home exercises are an effective treatment method that can be applied in the treatment of diseases whether it is given written or with video. Exercises reduce the pain of the patients and the fear of movement. (14) However, giving the exercises with video instead of the tables provides accurate and regular application of the exercises; therefore, home exercises with video is more effective than written exercises.(15) In our study, the relationship between the patient's attention level and the frequency of exercise were also investigated. However, the findings showed that the level of attention did not affect the frequency of exercise.

Limitations of the Research

Factors limiting our study include the number of patients included in the study, taking the heterogeneous patient population, not evaluating the pain in detail (frequency, time, etc.) and the inability of the study to be considered.

Author Contributions

Concept –.K.A.; Design – Ö.Ş; Analysis and/or Interpretation –.K.A.,J.Ö.A. .; Literature Review – Ö.Ş. Writing Manuscript –.K.A..; Critical Review -B.A.

Conflict of Interest

There is no conflict of interest by the authors.

Financial Disclosure

The authors declared that they did not receive financial support for this study.

References

1. Acar, M., Tonga, E., Ayyıldız, S. ve Balcı, B.(2014) Ankilozan Spondilitli Hastaların Egzersiz Kapasitesi, Nefes Darlığı, Göğüs Ekspansiyonu, Yaşam Kalitesi Ve Hastalık Aktivitesi Sonuçlarının İlişkisi. *Türk Toraks Derneği 17. Kongresi Sözlü Bildiriler.* p:6.4.

2. Alp, A., Cansever, Ş., Görgeç, N., Yurtkuran, M. ve Topsaç, T.(2009) Fiziksel Egzersizin Yaşlı Osteoporozlu Popülasyonda Denge ve Yaşam Kalitesi Üzerindeki Etkileri, *Türkiye Klinikleri Tıp Bilimleri Dergisi*, 29(3):687–695.

3. Ay,S., Doğan, Ş.K. ve Evcik, D.(2013) Diz Osteoartriti Olan Hastalarda Ev Egzersiz Programı Önermenin Etkili Bir Yolu Var mıdır? Randomize Kontrollü Bir Çalışma. *Türk Fiziksel Tıp ve Rehabilitasyon Dergisi*. 59:1–6.

4. Brown, D.J. & Lee, C.(2004). Grandmothers on the Move: Benefits,Barriers and Best Practice Intervantions for Physical Therapy in Older Women. In: Morris M, SCHOO A editors. *Optimizing Exercise and Physical Activity in Older People*. Edinburgh, Butterworth Heinemann, p.25–35.

5. Cheval,B., Tipura,E.,Burra,N., Frossard,J.,Chanal, J., Orsholits, D., Radel, R.& Boisgontier, M.P. et al.(2018) Avoiding Sedentary Behaviors Requires More Cortical Resources Than Avoiding Physical Activity: An EEG study. *J.Neuropsychologia*. 119: 68–80

6. Tunay, V.B., Baltacı, G. ve Atay, A.Ö. (2010) Hospital-Based versus Home-Based Proprioceptive and Strengthening Exercise Programs in Knee Osteoarthritis. Acta orthopaedica et traumatologica turcica (44) 4: 270–277.

7. Çatal, Ç., Alper, H. ve Şerbetçioğlu, E.(2014) KOAH Hastalarında Tele Pulmoner Rehabilitasyon İçin Kinect Temelli Ev Egzersiz Yazılımı, Ulusal Yazılım Mühendisliği Sempozyumu. *ODTÜ Kuzey Kıbrıs Kampüsü, KKTC, Bildiriler Kitabı*.1221: p: 96–101.

8. Schäfer, A.G.M., Zalpour, C., von Piekartz, H., Hall, T.M.&Paelke, V.(2018) The Efficacy of Electronic Health-Supported Home Exercise Interventions for Patients With Osteoarthritis of the Knee: Systematic Review. J Med Internet Res. 20(4): e152.

9. Karakaş, S., Eski, R. ve Başar, E.(1997) Türk kültürü için standardizasyonu yapılmış nöropsikolojik testler topluluğu: BİLNOT Bataryası. 32. Ulusal Noroloji Kongresi kitabı, Türk Nöroloji Dergisi. Ufuk Matbaası, İstanbul.

10. Wechsler, D. & Stone, C.P., (1945) Wechsler Memory Scale Manual. The Psychological Corporation. New York

11. Acar S, Savci S, Keskinoğlu P, Akdeniz B, Özpelit E, Özcan Kahraman B,Karadibak D, Sevinc C. Tampa Scale of Kinesiophobia for Heart Turkish Version Study: cross-cultural adaptation, exploratory factor analysis, and reliability. J Pain Res. 2016 Jun 23;9:445-51.

12. Pinar R. Reliability and construct validity of the SF-36 in Turkish cancer patients. Qual Life Res. 2005 Feb;14(1):259-64.

13. Ertekin, Ö., Özakbaş, S., İdiman, E., ve Algun Z.C.(2012).Multipl Skleroz Hastalarında Ev Egzersiz Programının Sonrasında Yaşam Kalitesi, Yorgunluk Ve Dengedeki İyileşmeler, Nöropsikiyatri Arşivi Dergisi, 49: 33–38

14. Nicolson, P.J.A., Hinman, R.S., Kasza, J. ve Bennell, K.L., (2018) Trajectories of Adherence to Home-Based Exercise Programs among People with Knee Osteoarthritis. *Osteoarthritis Cartilage.* 26(4):513–521.

15. Hong, J., Kong, H.J. & Yoon, H.J., (2018) Web-Based Telepresence Exercise Program for Community-Dwelling Elderly Women with a High Risk of Falling: Randomized Controlled Trial. JMIR M Health U Health. 6(5): 28

Leyla Ataş Balcı and Lütfü Hanoğlu

Effects of Dual-Task Training and Exercise-Cognitive Activity Combined Training on Gait Speed and Cognitive Skills in Older Adults: A Randomised Controlled Trial Study

Abstract: *Objective:* The purpose of this study was to compare the effect of dual-task and exercise-cognitive activity combined training on gait speed and cognitive skills in older adults.

Materials and Method: Forty-five volunteers were recruited. Participants were divided into 3 groups which consisted of i) a single-task performing balance and gait exercises ii) a dual-task training group performing cognitive activity with simultaneous balance and gait exercises and iii) an exercise-cognitive activity combined training group performing balance and gait activity asynchronously at different times during the same day. Gait speed under single-task and dual-task conditions were obtained at the onset and end of training period. Cognitive skills were assessed by Mini Mental, Stroop, Verbal Fluency, and Clock Drawing tests.

Results: All groups improved on gait speed under single-task condition. However, only cognitive activity performing groups showed a significant increase in gait speed under dual-task condition. Comparing pre- and post-intervention performances, dual-task and exercise-cognitive activity combined training groups showed a significant improvement in Stroop, Mini Mental, Verbal Fluency, and Clock Drawing test scores with respect to pre-intervention ($p<0.05$, paired t-test). The increase in Stroop and Verbal Fluency test scores post-intervention was significantly higher for exercise-cognitive activity combined training group when compared to dual-task training group ($p<0.05$). Exercise induced increase in gait speed correlated with improvements in cognitive skills for all groups ($p<0.05$).

Conclusion: The results suggest that daily living activities which require dual-tasks may be improved to a better extent by performing cognitive, balance, and gait activity training asynchronously at different times during the same day when compared with dual-task training.

Keywords: Aged, dual-task, executive function, falls, gait speed

Introduction

Cognitive skills and gait performance are known to deteriorate with aging, which is suggested to be associated with a decrease in the number of neurons and shrinkage of some cortical regions as well as hippocampus, substantia nigra, locus coeruleus, caudate nucleus, prefrontal cortex, and putamen (1, 2).

Prefrontal cortex is responsible for processing executive and cognitive functions related to reasoning, planning, sequencing, adapting to environmental stimuli, changing behaviors appropriately, and solving complex problems. These functions are also crucial for developing inner strategies (e.g., adaptation to ground changes and awareness of traffic signals) for avoiding accidents, which may cause morbidity and mortality at older ages (3).

Previous neuroimaging studies indicated a correlation between loss of gray and white matter volume in the frontal lobe and gait problems, cognitive disorders, and falls all of which constitute significant mortality risk in the elderly (4,5).

Most daily living activities involve simultaneous performance of two or more tasks such as walking and talking, referred to as a "dual-task". Performing gait under dual-tasking is accompanied with higher prefrontal cortex activity relative to normal gait (6).

In elderly, walking while simultaneously performing a motor or a cognitive task results in a higher increase in oxygenation of the prefrontal cortex, premotor cortex, and supplementary motor areas while it results in a decrease in gait speed compared to normal gait (7). It has been shown in many studies that dual-task deficits are caused by a decline in prefrontal cortical networks and prefrontal brain volume (8, 9).

Recent literature indicates that dual-task training, which combined strength, balance, and gait training with cognitive activities resulted in significantly better improvement in executive functions, dual-task costs of walking, and gait speed. In the elderly population, dual-task training was shown to be more effective in increasing gait speed and improving cognitive skills when compared to single-task training (10, 11). Although, dual-task training was shown to be more beneficial in improving gait speed and cognitive skills compared to gait and cognitive activities alone, the effects of performing cognitive activity, balance, and gait activity at different times during the day on cognitive skills and gait speed among elderly individuals have not been investigated. The purpose of this study was to compare the effect of dual-task training and exercise-cognitive activity combined training on gait speed and cognitive skills in healthy older adults.

Methods

Ethical Aspects of Research

The ethics committee of Istanbul Medipol University reviewed and approved the present study. All experiments were carried out in accordance with the Declaration of Helsinki. Written informed consent was obtained from all participants.

The Universe and Sample of Research

A total of 45 healthy older adults (73±4.62 years; 6 males and 38 females) participated in the study. Participants were over 65 years old, literate, had a fall incident during the year previous to their participation in the study. They were able to walk 10 m without any support and able to achieve a score of at least 24 in the Mini Mental Test (MMT). Individuals who had serious orthopedic problems, serious visual and auditory impairments, and neurological problems such as Stroke, Parkinson, or Alzheimer's disease were excluded from the study. The participants were randomly divided into 3 intervention groups: 1) a single-task group who performed only balance and gait exercises (1st group; n=15), 2) a dual-task training group who performed cognitive activities simultaneously with balance and gait exercises (2nd Group; n=15), and 3) an exercise-cognitive activity combined training group who performed balance, gait, and cognitive activities at different times during the same day (3rd Group; n=15). All participants accepted their group allocations.

Outcome Measurements

The following items were evaluated before and after intervention periods. All measurements were carried out by the same physiotherapist.

Gait Speed

Self-selected gait speed was measured under single- and dual-task conditions. Participants walked 10 m at their comfortable speed and time to completion was recorded by using a stopwatch. In the dual-task condition, participants were asked to produce words that began with the letter "K" while walking (12).

Cognitive Performance

Cognitive performance was quantified by MMT, Stroop Test, Verbal Fluency Tests (VFT), and Clock Drawing Test (CDT) scores.

MMT was applied to assess the general state of cognitive function. This assessment tool consists of orientation, registration, attention and calculation, recalling, language and visual constructive praxis categories that evaluate specific cognitive functions. Any score greater than or equal to 24 points indicates a normal cognition (13).

Stroop test evaluates the inhibition of inappropriate responses in executive functions (14). The Kaplan version of Stroop test was administered in the present study. This version of the Stroop test consists of three trials. Each trial is presented with a stimulus card with a presentation of 100 items. The first trial requires rapid naming of blocks of three different colors: red, green, and blue. The second trial requires rapid reading of the color words (red, green, and blue) printed in black ink. On third trial (the interference trial) the same words are presented, but ink color does not match with the word. Participants were instructed to name the color of the ink instead of reading the word. The total accurate numbers were measured.

VFT reflects sustained attention and monitors responses to prevent errors, including repetitions/perseverations. During this test, participants were asked to name many animals and generate words beginning with 'K', 'A', and 'S' letters as quick as possible in 1 minute. The total number of different animals named and words generated were recorded (15).

CDT is a test evaluating visuo-constructive and visuo-spatial skills, symbolic and conceptual representation, and organization and planning. Each participant was given a pre-drawn circle and asked to insert numbers. Then, participants were asked to place the clock hands to read '10 past 11'. In this study, the method by Freedman et al. (1994) was adopted to score CDT performances (16). This is a 13-point scoring system where 1 denotes very poor and 13 denotes the best performance. The scoring system consisted of 13 items. For each item, the scores were 0 or 1. Numbers, hands, and center were scored (16, 17).

Interventions

The participants received individualized training sessions three times a week for four weeks. The four-week training program consisting of balance and gait exercises was proven to be effective in improving balance function and dual-task performance in older adults (10) and was adapted for all intervention groups. The program included static balance exercises, static balance exercises, ball catching activities, and dynamic balance exercises. Static balance exercises were related to maintaining body stability (e.g., standing with eyes closed, standing legs open and closed, tandem standing, standing on foam surfaces, and standing on one leg) while throwing and catching a ball, weight shifting forward and backward on standing position, and keeping body stability while being disturbed by external perturbation. Dynamic balance exercises included tandem walking, walking backward, walking side to side, transferring from one chair to another, and sit to stand 5 times. Participants in the single-task group received 30 minutes of balance and gait exercises only, three times a week for 4 weeks.

Participants in Groups 2 and 3 practiced cognitive tasks while simultaneously or asynchronously performing balance and gait exercises. Examples of cognitive tasks have been described in detail elsewhere (10). At each week, participants performed different types of activities, which were designed to foster the abilities for planning, monitoring, and ordering, in addition to action inhibition and undesired processing. The cognitive tasks were associated with auditory attention (e.g., following verbal directions in which participants listened to news and they were asked to discriminate inappropriate parts), visual attention (participants spotted desired figures and/or words in a paper full of figures/Word, spotted the seven differences in pictures and were asked to name the color of the colored words), planning (performing a task placing words in order, such as days of the week, letters of the alphabet or placing sequences of a story in order), verbal fluency (verbal fluency with categorical and phonological constraints), simple mental math activities (addition, subtraction in two-digit numbers), and maze activities. Participants receiving dual-task training practiced 30 minutes of balance and gait exercises while simultaneously performing cognitive tasks, 3 times a week for 4 weeks while the participants in exercise-cognitive activity combined training group first practiced 30 minutes of cognitive activity, and then performed 30 minutes of balance and gait exercises after 5 minutes of resting with a frequency of 3 times a week for 4 weeks.

Statistical Analysis

The statistical analyses were carried out using IBM SPSS Statistics software, version 20 (SPSS, Chicago, IL, USA). The Shapiro-Wilk test was used to assess compliance of the data to the normal distribution. Comparison of outcome measurements between baseline and post-intervention within the groups was examined by Student's paired t-test and Wilcoxon test. The training effect on gait speed and verbal fluency among the groups was performed using ANOVA. The Scores of MMT, CDT, and Stroop test were not normally distributed. Therefore, Kruskal Wallis test was used to measure the training effects on MMT, CDT, and Stroop test among the groups (Bonferroni corrected Mann-Whitney U test). Pearson's Correlation test was used to analyze the relationship between the variables of gait speed and cognitive tests. The level of significance was set at 0.017 for Bonferroni corrected Mann-Whitney U test and 0.05 for others.

Results

Fifty-eight older adults were evaluated; 13 people did not meet the inclusion criteria (Fig. 1). Forty-five older adults completed the training program.

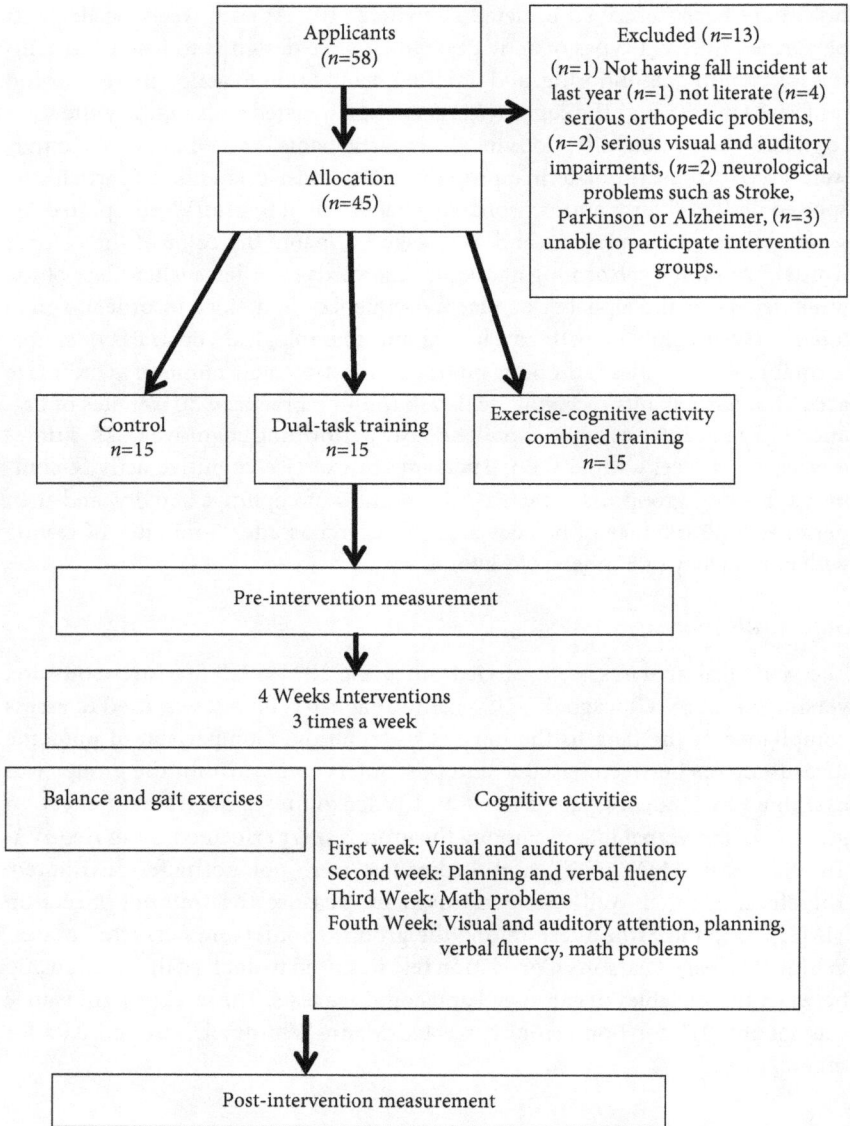

Fig. 1: The Flow Chart of the Study Participants

Baseline Characteristics

The mean age ± standard deviation (SD) of the participants was 70.73±4.62 years (range, 65–83y), and most of the participants was female (39 F, 6 M) (Tab. 1).

Effects of Interventions

There was a significant improvement in gait speed under single-task condition in all intervention groups after the training program (p<0.05) (Tab. 2). For gait speed under dual-task conditions, a significant improvement post-intervention was found in Groups 2 and 3 which received cognitive activities (p<0. 05) (Tab. 2). However, no statistically significant difference in gait speed improvement under dual-task conditions was found between Groups 2 and 3 (Tab. 3) (p>0.05) though the improvement in Group 3 was higher than Group 2 (Tab. 2).

There was a significant increase in the MMT and CDT scores after the interventions for individuals who received cognitive activities (Tab. 2) (p<0,017). Meanwhile, no significant changes were found at the single-task group after the intervention (Tab. 2). However, the participants who received exercise-cognitive activity combined training scored greater in MMT compared to dual-task training group (p<0.017) (Tab. 3). For Stroop test and VFT, there was a greater

Tab. 1: Baseline Characteristics of Participant's Data

Characteristics	Single-Task Training $n = 15$	Dual-Task Training $n = 15$	Exercise-Cognitive Activity Combined Training $n = 15$
Age	71.8 (4.1)	69.0 (5.1)	71.3 (4.2)
Gender	13 Female 2 Male	13 Female 2 Male	13 Female 2 Male
MMT	26.8 (1.6)	26.9 (1.3)	26.0 (1.0)
Single task gait speed (m/s)	0.78 (0.05)	0.77 (0.06)	0.76 (0.06)
Dual task gait speed (m/s)	0,63 (0,04)	0,64 (0,04)	0,62 (0,04)
Stroop	56.06 (1.90)	56.20 (1.14)	55.66 (1.79)
CDT	11.53 (1.24)	10.93 (1.43)	10.60 (1.35)
VFT/Animals	22.20 (4.61)	22.20 (5.90)	19.0 (3.29)
VFT/K, A, S	45.66 (7.48)	46.00 (9.60)	40.06 (6.19)

Values are mean (SD) MMT: Mini Mental Test CDT: Clock Drawing Test VFT: Verbal Fluency Tests

Tab. 2: Outcome Measures of Post-Training and Their Relative Change with Respect to Baseline Measurements for All Groups

	Single-Task Training n = 15			Dual-Task Training n = 15			Exercise-Cognitive Activity Combined Training n = 15		
	Post-training	Change	p	Post-training	Change	p	Post-training	Change	p
Single task gait speed (m/s)	0.8 (0.04)	0.03 (0.04)	0.007[a]	0.8 (0.07)	0.06 (0.05)	0.000[a]	0.9 (0.08)	0.1 (0.09)	0.000[a]
Dual task gait speed (m/s)	0.6 (0.05)	-0.002 (0.02)	0.733	0.7 (0.06)	0.08 (0.05)	0.000[a]	0.7 (0.05)	0.1 (0.05)	0.000[a]
MMT	27.13 (1.72)	0.33 (0.61)	0.055	27.53 (1.45)	0.60 (0.73)	0.003[b]	27.73 (0.96)	1.66 (0.97)	0.000[b]
Stroop	56.00 (1.77)	0.06 (0.88)	0.774	57.33 (1.29)	1.13 (0.63)	0.000[a]	57.40 (1.84)	1.73 (1.27)	0.000[a]
CDT	11.60 (1.45)	0.06 (0.79)	0.751	11.46 (0.99)	0.53 (0.74)	0.015[b]	11.93 (0.79)	1.33 (1.11)	0.003[b]
VFT/Animals	22.26 (5.36)	0.06 (2.25)	0.910	24.66 (7.03)	2.46 (1.50)	0.000[a]	23.46 (4.43)	4.46 (3.27)	0.000[a]
VFT/K, A, S	44.46 (7.28)	1.20 (2.98)	0.141	49.20 (9.41)	3.20 (2.04)	0.000[a]	41.86 (6.72)	1.80 (1.74)	0.001[a]

Values are mean (SD) MMT: Mini Mental Test CDT: Clock Drawing Test VFT: Verbal Fluency Test

[a] $p < 0.05$

[b] $p < 0.017$

Tab. 3: Comparison of Changes in Outcome Measures among Post and Pre Training Measurements among the 3 Groups

Variables	Groups	p
Single-task gait speed	1st-2nd	*0.000*[a]
	1st-3rd	*0.000*[a]
	2nd-3rd	*0.268*
Dual-task gait speed	1st-2nd	*0.000*[a]
	1st-3rd	*0.000*[a]
	2nd-3rd	*0.114*
MMT	1st-2nd	*0.317*
	1st-3rd	*0.000*[a]
	2nd-3rd	*0.002*[a]
VFT/Animals	1st-2nd	*0.006*[a]
	1st-3rd	*0.001*[a]
	2nd-3rd	*0.126*
VFT/K, A, S	1st-2nd	*0.000*[a]
	1st-3rd	*0.003*[a]
	2nd-3rd	*0.234*
Stroop	1st-2nd	*0.000*[a]
	1st-3rd	*0.000*[a]
	2nd-3rd	*0.182*
CDT	1st-2nd	*0.090*
	1st-3rd	*0.002*[a]
	2nd-3rd	*0.032*[a]

MMT: Mini Mental Test CDT: Clock Drawing Test VFT: Verbal Fluency Tests
[a] $p < 0.05$

improvement after training program in Groups 2 and 3 who received cognitive activities ($p < 0.05$) (Tab. 2). However, no significant difference in improvement was observed between dual-task training and exercise-cognitive activity combined training groups in Stroop test and VFT scores ($p > 0.05$) (Tab. 3). Nonetheless, although not statistically significant, participants in Group 3 had a greater improvement in cognitive skills.

Tab. 4 demonstrates the relationship between changes in gait speed and changes in cognitive performance scores over the training programs. Significant correlations were found between single-task gait speed and MMT ($r = 0.453$; $p = 0.002$), between single-task gait speed and VFT/Animals ($r = -0.573$; $p = 0.000$),

Tab. 4: The Relationship between Changes in Gait Speed and Changes in Cognitive Performance Scores over the Training Programs

Variable 1	Variable 2	r	p
Single-task gait speed	Stroop	0.467	*0.001*[a]
	CDT	0.436	*0.003*[a]
	VFT/Animals	0.573	*0.000*[a]
	VFT/K, A, S	0.282	*0.061*
	MMT	0.453	*0.002*[a]
Dual-task gait speed	Stroop	0.660	*0.000*[a]
	CDT	0.402	*0.006*
	VFT/Animals	0.553	*0.000*[a]
	VFT/K, A, S	0.534	*0.000*[a]
	MMT	0.535	*0.000*[a]

MMT: Mini Mental Test CDT: Clock Drawing Test VFT: Verbal Fluency Tests *r*: Pearson's correlation
[a] $p < 0.05$

between single-task gait speed and Stroop test (r=0.467; p=0.001), and between single-task gait speed and CDT (r=0.436; p=0.003) (p<0.05) (Tab. 4). A strong correlation was found between dual-task gait speed and MMT (r=0.535; p=0.000); between dual-task gait speed and VFT/Animals (r=0.553; p=0.000); between dual-task gait speed and VFT/K, A, S (r=0.534; p=0.000); between dual-task gait speed and Stroop test (r=0.660; p=0.000), and between dual-task gait speed and CDT (r=-0.402; p=0.006) (Tab. 4).

Discussion

In the present study, the effects of dual-task training and exercise-cognitive activity combined training on gait speed and cognitive performances were investigated in healthy older adults. Our results showed that both dual-task training and exercise-cognitive activity combined training improved gait speed and cognitive performances, while exercise-cognitive activity combined training resulted in greater improvement for cognitive performance.

Previous research indicated that performing cognitive activities simultaneously with balance, strengthening, and coordination enhance executive functions at elderly population more than single-task training (10, 11). In our findings, there was no difference in executive functions between the pre and post-intervention for the single-task training group. Executive functions of both dual-task and exercise-cognitive activity combined training groups were positively effected while exercise-cognitive activity combined training was observed to result in better improvement. Many studies showed similar results with our research where cognitive activities performed in addition to balance, strengthening, and walking activities were reported to improve cognitive performance more than performing balance, strengthening, and walking activities only (18, 19). As such, Law et al. (2014) declared that the combination of cognitive activity and physical exercises increases cognitive performance in elderly on their systematic review (18).

Gait speed under single-task and dual-task conditions of the dual-task training group increased by 0.06 m/s and 0.09 m/s while those of the exercise-cognitive activity combined training group increased by 0.18 m/s and 0.12 m/s, respectively. However, both dual task training and exercise-cognitive activity combined training programs were equally effective in improving gait speed under single- and dual-task conditions. These findings suggest that older adults are able to improve their gait performance under dual-task conditions by cognitive task included training programs. According to previous studies, the efficient integration and coordination between the two tasks is crucial for improving dual-task performance (10). This may explain the improvement in dual-task performance after dual-task training. Alternatively, according to the study of Ruthruff et al. (2006), practicing only one task at a time allows participants to automatize the performance of individual tasks. Thus, participants can perform more rapid movements by decreasing the demand required for performing dual task (20). It is possible that participants in our study who received exercise-cognitive activity combined training could perform a faster gait speed under dual-task conditions by training of balance and cognitive skills separately.

Correlation analysis revealed exercise training induced changes in cognitive performances and gait speed. This association supported the statement that decrease in gait speed can be an indicator of possible cognitive problems in the future (21, 22).

Limitations

The following limitations have to be acknowledged. First, sample size of the present study was small (number of participants at each group was 15). Second, the majority of participants in the study were women, which may introduce bias in resembling a universal population in statistical analyses. Third, the amount of improvement recorded in the exercise-cognitive activity combined training group could be the consequence of receiving a longer treatment (60 minutes) compared to single task training and dual-task training groups (which had 30 minutes intervention). Last, our intervention period was short. For future investigations, it will be interesting to apply the same protocol on gender balanced groups with a greater sample size.

Conclusion

To the best of our knowledge, this is the first study to show the comparison of the effects of single-task, dual-task, and exercise-cognitive activity combined training on cognitive performances and gait speed in old people. Despite the increase of gait speed and cognitive performances after dual-task training, exercise-cognitive activity combined training was significantly more effective in improving cognitive and motor performances. Furthermore, the prefrontal adaptations were correlated with improved performance in executive functions and gait speed. The practical importance of this study is for daily living activities which require dual-task performance such as walking while talking and crossing streets might be more facilitated by exercise-cognitive activity combined training. Future investigations should focus on applying a similar experimental protocol on a greater population consisting of gender balanced groups while paying attention to living the same dose of training for each intervention group.

Acknowledgments

The authors wish to thank Assoc. Prof. Hanefi Ozbek for his help relating to the statistical analyses.

Disclosure Statement

Conflict of interest: The authors declare no conflict of interest.
Financial disclosure: The authors declare no financial support for the study.

References

1. Atkinson, H.H., Rosano, C., Simonsick, E.M., et al. (2007). Cognitive Function, Gait Speed Decline, and Comorbidities: The Health, Aging and Body Composition Study. *J Gerontol A Biol Sci Med Sci.*, 62: 844–850.
2. Holtzer, R., Epstein, N., Mahoney, J.R., Izzetoglu, M., Blumen, H.M. (2014). Neuroimaging of Mobility in Aging: A Targeted Review. *J Gerontol A Biol Sci Med Sci.*, 69: 1375–1388.

3. Yogev-Seligmann, G., Hausdorff, J.M., Giladi, N. (2008). The Role of Executive Function and Attention in Gait. *Mov Disord.*,; 23: 329–342; quiz 472.

4. Rosano, C., Studenski, S.A., Aizenstein, H.J., Boudreau, R.M., Longstreth, W.T., Newman, A.B. (2012). Slower Gait, Slower Information Processing and Smaller Prefrontal Area in Older Adults. *Age Ageing*, 41: 58–64.

5. Walshe, E.A., Patterson, M.R., Commins, S., Roche, R.A. (2015). Dual-Task and Electrophysiological Markers of Executive Cognitive Processing in Older Adult Gait and Fall-Risk. *Front Hum Neurosci.*, 9: 200.

6. Mirelman, A., Maidan, I., Bernad-Elazari, H., et al. (2014). Increased Frontal Brain Activation During Walking While Dual Tasking: An fNIRS Study in Healthy Young Adults. *J Neuroeng Rehabil.*, 11: 85.

7. Lu, C.F., Liu, Y.C., Yang, Y.R., Wu, Y.T.,Wang, R.Y. (2015). Maintaining Gait Performance by Cortical Activation during Dual-Task Interference: A Functional Near-Infrared Spectroscopy Study. *PLoS One*, 10: e0129390.

8. Raz, N., Lindenberger, U., Rodrigue, K.M., et al. (2005). Regional Brain Changes in Aging Healthy Adults: General Trends, Individual Differences and Modifiers. *Cereb Cortex.*, 15: 1676–1689.

9. Beurskens, R., &Bock, O. (2012). Age-Related Deficits of Dual-Task Walking: A Review. *Neural Plast.*, 131–608.

10 .Silsupadol, P., Shumway-Cook, A., Lugade, V., et al. (2009). Effects of Single-Task versus Dual-Task Training on Balance Performance in Older Adults: A Double-Blind, Randomized Controlled trial. *Arch Phys Med Rehabil.*, 90: 381–387.

11. Plummer, P., Zukowski, L.A., Giuliani, C., Hall, A.M., Zurakowski, D. (2015). Effects of Physical Exercise Interventions on Gait-Related Dual-Task Interference in Older Adults: A Systematic Review and Meta-Analysis. *Gerontology*, 62: 94–117.

12. Shubert, T.E., Schrodt, L.A.,Mercer, V.S., Busby-Whitehead, J., Giuliani, C.A. (2006). Are Scores on Balance Screening Tests Associated with Mobility in Older Adults? *J Geriatr Phys Ther.*, 29: 35–39.

13. Keskinoğlu, P., Uçku, R., Yener, G. (2008). Pretest Results of the Revised Standardized Mini Mental Examination Test in Community Dwelling Elderly. *Journal of Neurological Sciences*, 25: 18–24.

14. Kang, C.,Lee, G.J., Yi, D., et al. (2013). Normative Data for Healthy Older Adults and an Abbreviated Version of the Stroop test. *Clin Neuropsychol.*, 27: 276–289.

15. Stein, J., Luppa, M., Brähler, E., König, H.H., Riedel-Heller, S.G. (2010). The Assessment of Changes in Cognitive Functioning: Reliable Change

Indices for Neuropsychological Instruments in the Elderly - a Systematic Review. *Dement Geriatr Cogn Disord.*, 29: 275–286.

16. Freedman, M., Leach, L., Kaplan, E., et al. (1994). Clock Drawing: A Neuropsychological Analysis. *Oxford University Press*: New York.

17. Ricci, M., Pigliautile, M.,D'Ambrosio, V., et al. (2016). The Clock Drawing Test as a Screening Tool in Mild Cognitive Impairment and Very Mild Dementia: A New Brief Method of Scoring and Normative Data in the Elderly. *Neurol Sci.*, 37: 867–873.

18. Law, L.L., Barnett, F., Yau, M.K., Gray, M.A. (2014). Effects of Combined Cognitive and Exercise Interventions on Cognition in Older Adults with and without Cognitive Impairment: A Systematic Review. *Ageing Res Rev.*, 15: 61–75.

19. van het Reve, E., &de Bruin, E.D. (2014). Strength-Balance Supplemented with Computerized Cognitive Training to Improve Dual Task Gait and Divided Attention in Older Adults: A Multicenter Randomized-Controlled Trial. *BMC Geriatr.*, 14: 134.

20. Ruthruff, E., Van Selst, M., Johnston, J.C., Remington, R. (2006). How Does Practice Reduce Dual-Task Interference: Integration, Automatization, or Just Stage-Shortening? *Psychol Res.*, 70: 125–142.

21. Deshpande, N., Metter, E.J., Bandinelli, S., Guralnik, J., Ferrucci, L. (2009). Gait Speed under Varied Challenges and Cognitive Decline in Older Persons: A Prospective Study. *Age Ageing*, 38: 509–514.

22. Callisaya, M.L., Blizzard, C.L., Wood, A.G., Thrift, A.G., Wardill, T., Srikanth, V.K. (2015). Longitudinal Relationships Between Cognitive Decline and Gait Slowing: The Tasmanian Study of Cognition and Gait. *J Gerontol A Biol Sci Med Sci.*, 70: 1226–1232.

Leyla Ataş Balcı, Hazal Öksüz, Çiçek Duman, and
Hasan Kerem Alptekin

The Attitudes of Physiotherapy and Rehabilitation Students towards Elderly

Abstract: *Objective:* The rapid increase in aging shifted the healthcare professionals to work more frequently with elderly. To improve healthcare services, positive attitudes and behaviours of health professionals such as physiotherapists towards older people keep importance. The purpose of this study was to determine the attitudes of physiotherapy and rehabilitation students towards the elderly.

Material and Method: The Turkish version of UCLA-GA Scale was used to evaluate attitudes towards older people among 265 students of Bahçeşehir University, Department of Physiotherapy and Rehabilitation in Istanbul in Turkey. Also socio-demographical characteristics of the students were obtained with a structured questionnaire.

Results: The mean total UCLA-GAS scores of the participants were 47.28±5.68. Female participants were determined to have a more positive attitude towards older people, compared to male students (p<0.01). Especially, female participants had greater scores in compassion and resource distribution sub-dimensions (p<0.05). The participants who visited nursing homes had more positive attitudes towards older people (p<0.01). The participants whose mother had undergraduate degree significantly showed a more positive attitude towards older people, compared to participants whose mother had primary school or high school degrees (p<0.05).

Conclusion: In conclusion, positive attitudes of physiotherapy and rehabilitation students towards elderly could be affected by gender, visiting nursing homes and maternal educational status.

Keywords: Aged, Aging, Attitude of Health Personnel, Behaviour, Students

Introduction

Population ageing is the most significant social changes of the twenty-first century. With gradual improvement in healthcare delivery services, life expectancy and the percentage of the elderly population have increased. According to data from World Population Prospects: the 2017 Revision, the number of persons aged 60 years or over is expected to more than double by 2050 (1). Also, according to official reports of the Statistic Institute of Turkey (2015), it has been estimated that the number of people aged ≥ 65 years will increase to 20.8 % by 2050 (2). These demographic transformations require shifting the global focus to medical needs of elderly population.

Considering the needs and problems of the elderly is an important social issue. The elderly population tends to have a higher prevalence of chronic diseases, physical disabilities, mental illnesses requiring more complex medical treatments and multiple prescription of medications (3). One of the limitations in providing high quality healthcare services to the elderly is negative attitudes, which may lead decrease of efficiency of the healthcare services (4). New report by WHO (2015) claimed that negative or ageist attitudes towards older people are widespread and negatively affect health of elderly individuals (5) .

Physiotherapists, the members in the team of healthcare services, frequently work with older people to improve functional performance, participation of daily living activities, and quality of life. As a part of geriatric rehabilitation, physiotherapists not only use therapeutic approaches, but also encourage older individuals to live active and maintaining functional status (6). For planning the goal-directed rehabilitation programs, communication with elderly is crucial which may be affected by negative attitudes.

Previous researches demonstrated that there are many factors that affect the attitudes of healthcare professionals towards older individuals including age, gender, education, living with elderly individuals and area of practice (7). The attitudes of health sciences students such as nursing, medical and pharmacy students towards older individuals are also important and have been assessed by many previous studies from different countries (8, 9). These studies revealed that healthcare students have difficulty in understanding and empathizing of elderly which will negatively impact their attitudes towards the elderly. Previous researches from Turkey showed contrast findings as the students from health sciences faculties commonly showed positive attitudes towards elderly individuals (10, 11). However these studies commonly recommended to increase of positive attitudes to geriatric population and to add gerontology or geriatric rehabilitation courses to academic education. These studies mainly focused on the effects of gender, age, educational status, working experiences and living with elderly on the attitudes that showed different results (10, 11).

Previous studies, comparing the attitudes of physiotherapy and other students of health sciences towards the elderly, found more positive attitude among the physiotherapy students (12, 13). However, the attitudes of physiotherapy students towards elderly people can change, depend on gender, having attendant to geriatric rehabilitation training or courses and living with older people. The present study aimed to investigate the attitudes of physiotherapy and rehabilitation students of the Faculty of Health Sciences of the Bahçeşehir University towards elderly. Further, this study aimed to identify the relationship of parental educational status and socio-economic status of physiotherapy and rehabilitation students with attitudes towards elderly.

Materials and Method

Design and Sample

This descriptive study was conducted on students of the Faculty of Health Sciences of the Bahçeşehir University between April and June 2018, in Istanbul. A total of 265 students in the physiotherapy and rehabilitation departments (first-to-fourth grades) voluntarily participated in this study. Signed informed consent was obtained from all students. The ethics committee of Bahçeşehir University approved the study, which was conducted according to the Declaration of Helsinki.

Data Collection Method and Instruments

The students completed the self-administered questionnaires. Socio-demographical characteristics of the students were obtained with a structured questionnaire. The socio-demographical form was included questions about age, gender, longest lived residence, parental educational status, income status, living with elderly people and visiting nursing homes.

The University of California, Los Angeles Geriatrics Attitudes Scale (UCLA-GAS) was used to evaluate attitudes towards elderly. This scale was developed by Reuben et al. (1998), and validity and reliability studies were performed by Sahin et al. (2012) (14, 15). The UCLA-GAS is a 14-item scale using 5-point Likert-scale responses indicating whether the respondent agrees or disagrees with the statement (The choices: 'strongly disagree', 'disagree', 'neutral', 'agree' and 'strongly agree'). On the items containing positive attitudes towards the elderly, scores range from 1 to 5, for items with negative attitudes, the scoring scheme is reversed. The survey has four dimensions: social values, medical care, compassion and resource distribution. The total score is obtained by combining all four dimensions. The UCLA-GAS scores range from 14 to 70, with higher scores indicating a more positive attitude. Average scores can also be calculated, with averages of 1 to 2 indicating negative scores, 3 indicating neutral scores and 4 to 5 indicating positive scores.

Statistical Analysis

The analyses were carried out using IBM SPSS Statistics software, version 20 (SPSS, Chicago, IL, USA). The level of significance was set at $p < 0.05$. Data were evaluated using descriptive statistics (number, percentage, distribution, average, standard deviation). Relationships between the scores obtained from the UCLA-GAS and socio-demographic characteristics of the participants were evaluated using Student's t-test and the one way ANOVA. Further Post-Hoc LSD analyses were performed to determine the relationship between sub-dimensions scores and socio-demographic characteristics of participants.

Results

A total of 215 physiotherapy students aged between 19 and 27 years (20.9±1.5 years; 158 female and 57 male) participated in the present study. 35.3 % of the students were in 1st grade and 73.5 % of them were female. Socio-demographic characteristics of the physiotherapy students are demonstrated in Tab. 1. Most of the participants were living in the province (64.2 %). Three mothers of participants had no education in the school (1.4 %). The highest percentage of parental educational status was in the high school degree, 33 % for mothers and %40.9 for father's educational status, respectively. Most of participants had income level between '1000' and '2000' TRY. Most of students do not live with an older individual (91.6 %). However 60.9 % of the students have been visited nursing homes (Tab. 1).

The mean total UCLA-GAS scores of the participants were 47.28±5.68 (min: 26, max: 63). Mean scores of four dimensions were as follows: social values: 6.16±1.54; medical care: 11.60±2.56; compassion: 15.33±2.88; resource distribution: 14.17±2.40. Female participants were determined to have a more positive attitude towards older people, compared to male students (p<0.01) (Tab. 2). Especially there was strong relationship between gender and compassion scores (p<0.04); between gender and resource distribution (p<0.05) (Tab. 3). Female participants had greater scores in compassion and resource distribution sub dimensions (Tab. 3).

The participants who visited nursing homes had more positive attitudes towards older people (p<0.01) (Tab. 2). There was a significant relationship between resource distribution scores and visiting nursing homes. Although there were no significant relationship between total UCLA-GAS scores and grade of education, parental educational status, income level, longest living residence and living with an older individual, there was a significant relationship between compassion scores and the educational status (p<0.01) (Tab. 3). The participants whose mother had undergraduate degree significantly showed a more positive attitude towards older people, compared to participants whose mother had primary school or high school degrees (Tab. 3).

Tab. 1: Socio-Demographic Characteristics of the Physiotherapy Students

Characteristics		n	%
Gender	Female	158	73.5
	Male	57	26.5
Grade	1	76	35.3
	2	55	25.6
	3	69	32.1
	4	15	7.0
Income status	0–500	36	16.7
	500–1000	53	24.7
	1000–2000	61	28.4
	2000–3000	32	14.9
	3000-above	33	15.3
Longest living residence	Village	4	1.9
	Town	1	0.5
	District	72	33.5
	Province	138	64.2
Educational status of mother	None	3	1.4
	Primary school	41	19.1
	Secondary school	29	13.5
	High school	71	33.0
	Undergraduate	50	23.3
	Postgraduate	21	9.8
Educational status of father	None	0	0
	Primary school	30	14.0
	Secondary school	24	11.2
	High school	88	40.9
	Undergraduate	54	25.1
	Postgraduate	19	8.8
Presence of living with elderly people	Yes	18	8.4
	No	197	91.6
Visiting the nursing home	Yes	131	60.9
	No	84	39.1

Discussion

The dramatic increase in average life expectancy during the 20th century, shifted healthcare services to focus on healthy aging approaches. Since the chronic diseases are more commonly seen in older ages, needs of healthcare professionals like physiotherapists will increase. The present study aimed to investigate the attitudes of physiotherapy students towards elderly. Also, the current study demonstrated the relationship of parental educational status and socio-economic

Tab. 2: Distribution of UCLA-GAS Total Scores, According to Their Socio-demographic Characteristics

Characteristics		UCLA Total		
		Mean (SD)	t/f	p
Gender	Female	48.05 (5.58)	**3.37**[x]	***0.01****
	Male	45.15 (5.46)		
Grade	1	47.55 (6.15)	0.31	*0.81*
	2	47.18 (5.27)		
	3	46.86 (5.58)		
	4	48.20 (5.50)		
Income status	0–500	47.16 (5.88)	1.02	*0.39*
	500–1000	47.18 (5.61)		
	1000–2000	46.68 (6.21)		
	2000–3000	46.87 (4.36)		
	3000-above	49.06 (5.66)		
Longest living residence	Village	45.00 (2.58)	0.24	*0.69*
	District	47.48 (5.72)		
	Province	47.24 (5.76)		
Educational status of mother	None	42.33 (4.04)	1.62	*0.15*
	Primary school	45.85 (5.88)		
	Secondary school	46.79 (6.28)		
	High school	47.88 (5.15)		
	Undergraduate	48.40 (5.33)		
	Postgraduate	46.76 (6.64)		
Educational status of father	None	0.00 (0.00)	0.82	*0.51*
	Primary school	46.50 (6.64)		
	Secondary school	46.29 (4.99)		
	High school	47.70 (5.11)		
	Undergraduate	46.94 (5.88)		
	Postgraduate	48.78 (6.86)		
Presence of living with elderly people	Yes	47.66 (3.10)	0.29[bold]	*0.76*
	No	47.24 (5.86)		
Visiting the nursing home	Yes	48.05 (5.68)	**2.50**[bold]	***0.01****
	No	46.08 (5.51)		

*p<0.05 f: One Way ANOVA Test
[x]t: Student's *t*-Test

Tab. 3: Distribution of Scores of Participants According to the Four Dimensions of UCLA-GAS

Characteristics		Social values			Medical care			Compassion			Resource distribution		
		Mean (SD)	t/f	p	Mean (SD)	t/f	p	Mean (SD)	t/f	p	Mean (SD)	t/f	p
Gender	Female[a]	6.20 (1.57)	0.51[x]	0.60	11.65 (2.51)	0.40[x]	0.68	15.67 (2.66)	2.88[x]	0.04[α]	14.52 (2,36)	3.68[x]	0.00[α]
	Male[b]	6.07 (1.85)			11.49 (2.69)			14.40 (3.28)			13,19 (2,24)		
Grade	1	6.07 (1.83)	0.53	0.66	11.90 (2.48)	0.96	0.41	15.15(2.95)	0.35	0.78	14.40 (2.49)		0.40
	2	6.36 (1.68)			11.43 (2.75)			15.67(2.80)			13.70 (2.24)		
	3	6.05 (1.42)			11.30 (2.41)			15.27(3.04)			14.23 (2.44)		
	4	6.40 (1.59)			12.13 (2.87)			15.26 (2.08)			14.40 (2.29)		
Income status	0–500	6.27 (1.46)	0.53	0.70	11.44 (2.18)	0.82	0.51	15.33 (3.24)	1.24	0.29	14.11 (2.62)	0.88	0.47
	500–1000	6.03 (1.64)			11.60 (2.62)			15.58 (2.47)			13.96 (2.49)		
	1000–2000	6.26 (1.93)			11.62 (2.67)			14.68 (3.15)			14.11 (2.15)		
	2000–3000	5.87 (1.51)			11.12 (2.67)			15.90 (2.71)			13.96 (2.50)		
	3000–above	6.36 (1.41)			12.24 (2.52)			15.57 (2.68)			14.87 (2.36)		
Longest living residence	Village	6.75 (1.50)	0.22	0.87	11.00 (1.82)	0.22	0.88	13.25 (3.40)	0.81	0.48	14.00 (2.16)	0.31	0.81
	District	6.22 (1.61)			11.77 (2.13)			15.37 (2.90)			14.11 (2.31)		
	Province	6.12 (1.68)			11.53 (2.78)			15.36 (2.87)			14.22 (2.47)		
Educational status of mother	None[c]	5.66 (3.21)	1.55	0.17	12.66 (2.51)	1.39	0.22	12.00 (3.46)	2.76	0.01[β]	12.00 (1.00)	0.6	0.65
	Primary school[d]	5.78 (1.38)			11.46 (2.66)			14.63 (3.17)			13.97(2.63)		
	Secondary school[e]	6.03 (1.82)			11.44 (2.01)			15.06 (2.71)			14.00 (2.22)		
	High school[f]	6.22 (1.47)			11.19 (2.35)			15.31 (3.51)			14.28 (2.60)		
	Undergraduate[g]	6.64 (1.39)			12.36 (2.50)			16.18 (2.43)			14.34 (2.29)		
	Postgraduate[h]	5.85 (2.47)			11.57 (3.55)			15.00 (2.46)			14.33 (1.87)		

(continued on next page)

Tab. 3: (continued)

Characteristics		Social values (Mean (SD))	test	p	Medical care (Mean (SD))	test	p	Compassion (Mean (SD))	test	p	Resource distribution (Mean (SD))	test	p
Educational status of father	None	0.00 (0.00)	0.97	0.42	0.00 (0.00)	1.31	0.26	0.00 (0.00)	1.91	0.10	0.00 (0.00)	0.42	0.78
	Primary school	5.83 (1.36)			11.63 (2.44)			14.60 (3.70)			14.43 (2.75)		
	Secondary school	6.58 (1.69)			10.95 (1.94)			15.08 (2.70)			13.66 (2.23)		
	High school	6.07 (1.63)			11.42 (2.45)			15.94 (2.35)			14.26 (2.47)		
	Undergraduate	6.18 (1.51)			11.85 (2.58)			14.85 (3.12)			14.05 (2.19)		
	Postgraduate	6.52 (2.31)			12.57 (3.56)			15.36 (2.94)			14.31 (2.40)		
Presence of living with elderly people	Yes	6.38 (1.37)	0.59ˣ	0.55	11.38 (1.78)	0.38ˣ	0.70	15.05 (2.71)	0.42ˣ	0.66	14.83 (1.82)	1.22ˣ	0.22
	No	6.14 (1.67)			11.62 (2.62)			15.36 (2.90)			14.11 (2.44)		
Visiting the nursing home	Yes	6.29 (1.66)	1.36ˣ	0.17	11.79 (2.63)	1.32ˣ	0.18	15.40 (2.80)	0.44ˣ	0.66	14.56 (2.35)	3.04ˣ	0.03*
	No	5.97 (1.61)			11.32 (2.43)			15.22 (3.02)			13.55 (2.36)		

a post hoc LSD: a>b
β post hoc LSD: g>d; g >f
* p<0.05 f: One Way ANOVA Test
ˣ: Student's t-Test

status of physiotherapy and rehabilitation students with attitude towards elderly people.

The effect of gender on attitudes of healthcare students towards elderly has been researched by many studies (9, 10, 12). Because of the cultural changes, there were differences in attitudes towards elderly between Turkish culture and other countries (16). The previous studies from Turkey that determined the relationship of gender with attitudes of healthcare students towards elderly commonly showed that female students have more positive attitudes compared with male students (12, 17, 18). The present study also demonstrated similar results with studies from Turkey. Especially female students had greater scores in compassion and resource distribution items in the present study. There are several reason which might explain why female students showed greater positive attitudes towards elderly. Firstly, since, Turkey is a traditional society, Turkish people respect to the experiences and knowledge of elderly individuals. Also, females have caregiving and nurturing roles in the Turkish society (19). Secondly, most of the participants were female in the present study.

The students having similar intelligence level may have different expression and behaviour to same events due to socio-economic and educational status of their parents (20). Mothers have the greatest impact on the development and education of children. Previous researches have determined that increases in maternal education are associated with improved problem solving ability, increases in student's cognitive scores, decrease in behavioural problems, sexism and conservatism, cigarette and drug abuse (20–23). The present study demonstrated that the students whose mother graduated from university got greater scores in compassion items compared with students whose mother was graduated from primary school or high school. The higher the mothers' education level, the less the negative attitudes towards elderly individuals. Also, these results may change in the countries, on which fathers and mothers are equal in caregiving of children. Future studies are required to investigate whether these improvements remain valid in studies designed with larger and more homogenous sample groups of participants and in the different societies.

Recent decades have demonstrated significant changes in family dynamic due to rapid changes in the socioeconomic structures. The traditional model of caring elderly at home is changing to the modern model as institute them in the nursing homes (24). According to Elderly Care Services Report of Turkey (2017), 24,020 elderly individuals were cared in the private or state nursing homes by July 2016 (25). In the current study, visiting nursing homes by students was shown to be effective for developing positive attitudes towards the elderly. As a result, we thought that visiting nursing homes periodically should be encouraged by universities to raise awareness, to establish relationship between students and elderly, and to improve attitudes towards elderly people.

Previous findings showed that attitudes of physiotherapy students towards older adults were generally more positive than neutral (12, 13). The possible factors effects the attitudes, beliefs and knowledge of physiotherapy students were including age, clinical exposure and attendance to geriatric or gerontology courses, and contact with older adults (12, 13). They demonstrated that the attitudes and behaviour of the physiotherapy students may vary related to attendance of geriatric rehabilitation courses. Similarly, the current findings showed that the mean UCLA-GAS scores were 47.28±5.68 which determined that physiotherapy and rehabilitation students have positive attitudes towards elderly. The factors that may be related with positive scores could be maternal education status and visiting nursing homes. However the attendance of geriatric courses have not been evaluated. Further studies could be performed to determine whether the physiotherapy and rehabilitation students attending to geriatric rehabilitation courses show more positive scores.

Conclusion

In conclusion, attitudes of physiotherapy and rehabilitation students towards the elderly may change according to gender, visiting nursing homes or maternal educational status. Therefore, to improve attitudes to elderly, the visiting of nursing homes must be reinforced. Additionally, females should be educated not only to improve their attitudes towards the elderly, but also to shape positive behaviour in their children. Further suggestions the university curriculums have to establish awareness of elderly health and as role models, the lecturer of the physiotherapy and rehabilitation departments should encourage their students for more contact with elderly individuals.

Limitations

There are some limitations needed to be acknowledged. This study evaluated attitudes of only one university's physiotherapy and rehabilitation students towards elderly; hence, the results cannot be generalised to all physiotherapy and rehabilitation students in Turkey or in other countries. Future studies are required to investigate whether these improvements remain valid in studies designed with larger and more homogenous sample groups of participants and in the different universities and different countries. The attendance of geriatric courses have not been evaluated in the current study. Further studies could be performed to determine the effects of attending to geriatric courses or giving geriatric education on the attitudes towards elderly among the physiotherapy and rehabilitation students.

Disclosure Statement

We would like to state that the above-mentioned manuscript has not been published elsewhere, has not been accepted for publication elsewhere or under editorial review for publication elsewhere. The authors declare no conflict of interest.

References

1. United Nations, Department of Economic and Social Affairs, Population Division. (2017). World Population Prospects: The 2017 Revision, Key Findings and Advance Tables. Working Paper No. ESA/P/WP/248.

2. Turkish Statistical Institute. (2017). İstatistiklerle Yaşlılar, Sayı: 27595. http://www.tuik.gov.tr/PreHaberBultenleri.do?id=27595 (19.11.2018).

3. Shrivastava, S. R., Shrivastava, P. S., & Ramasamy, J. (2013). Health-care of Elderly: Determinants, Needs and Services. *International Journal of Preventive Medicine*, 4(10), 1224–1225.

4. Doherty, M., Mitchell, E.A., &O'Neill, S. (2011). Attitudes of Healthcare Workers towards Older People in a Rural Population: A Survey Using the Kogan Scale. *Nursing Research and Practice*, vol. 2011: 7

5. World Health Organization. (2015) . *World Report on Ageing and Health. World Health Organization.* Geneva. Retrieved from http://www.who.int/iris/handle/10665/186463.

6. İnal S.H., Subasi, F. (2013). Geriatric Rehabilitation. In: *Horizons in Geriatric Care*, Işık, A.T., Mas, M.R., Karan, M.A., & Grosberg, G.T. (Eds.). Chapter 15, pp.287–317, Nova Science Publishers, New York.

7. Arani, M.M., Aazami, S., Azami, M. Borji, M. (2017). Assessing Attitudes toward Elderly among Nurses Working in the City of Ilam, International *Journal of Nursing Sciences*, Volume 4, Issue 3.

8. Deasey, D., Kable, A., Jeong, S. (2014). Influence of Nurses' Knowledge of Ageing and Attitudes towards Older People on Therapeutic Interactions in Emergency Care: A Literature Review. *Australas. J Ageing*; 33(4): 229–36.

9. Turan, E., Yanardag, M., Metintas, S. (2015). Attitudes of students of health sciences towards the older persons. *Nurse Educ Today*; S0260-6917(15): 00281–6.

10. Kalaycı, I., Özbek Yazıcı, S., Özkul, M., Helvacı, G. (2017). Sağlık Çalışanları ve Öğrencilerinin Yaşlılara Yönelik Tutumları: Sistematik Derleme. *Adnan Menderes Üniversitesi, Sağlık Bilimleri Fakültesi Dergisi*, 1(1): 21–30.

11. Türgay, A.S, Şahin, S., Şenuzun Aykar, S., Sari, S., Badir, A., &Canli Özer, A. (2015). Atitudes of Turkish Nursing Students toward Elderly People, *European Geriatric Medicine*, 6(3): 267–270.

12. Bakırhan, S., Özkeskin, M., Aktar Reyhanioğlu, D., & Gülpinar, D. (2017). Analysis of the Attitudes and Approaches of the Physiotherapy and Rehabilitation Students towards the Elderly. *Turkish Journal of Geriatrics/ Türk Geriatri Dergisi*, 20(2): 125–134.

13. Kalu, E. M., Abaraogu, O.U., & Norman, K.E. (2018). Do Physiotherapy Students Demonstrate Ageist Attitude? A Scoping Review of Literature. *Physical & Occupational Therapy in Geriatrics*, 36:1, 72–89.

14. Reuben, D.B., Lee, M., Davis, J.W. Jr., Eslami, M.S., Osterweil, D.G., Melchiore, S., &Weintraub, N.T. (1998). Development and Validation of a Geriatrics Attitudes Scale for Primary Care Residents. *J Am Geriatr Soc*; 46(11): 1425–1430.

15. Sahin, S., Mandıracıoğlu, A., Tekin, N., Senuzun, F., Akcicek, F. (2012). Attitudes toward the Elderly among the Health Care Providers: Reliability and Validity of Turkish Version of the UCLA Geriatrics Attitudes (UCLA-GA) Scale. *Arch Gerontol Geriatr*; 55(1): 205–209.

16. Özmen, S.Y. (2013). Place of Old People in Turkish Culture and the Changing Position of Elderliness in Media. *International and Quarterly Journal of Cultural Studies*; 25: 110–119.

17. Soyuer, F., Unalan, D., Guleser, N., Elmalı, F. (2010). Attitudes of Students towards Ageism and the Relations with Various Demographic Variables. *Mersin Univ Sağlık Bilim Journal*, 3(2): 20–25.

18. Özbek Yazıcı, S. Kalaycı, I., Esin, K.,Tekin, A. (2015).Yaşlı bakım programı öğrencilerinin yaşlı ayrımcılığına ilişkin tutumları. *Yaşlı Sorunları Araştırma Dergisi*; 8(2):77–87.

19. Ayoglu, F.N., Kulakcı, H., Ayyıldız, T.K.,Aslan, G.K., Veren, F. (2013). Attitudes of Turkish Nursing and Medical Students toward Elderly People. *J Transcult Nurs*; 25(3): 241–248.

20. Eskicumali, A., Eroğlu, E. (2014). Ailenin Sosyo-Ekonomik ve Eğitim Düzeyleri ile Çocuklarin Problem Çözme Yetenekleri Arasindaki İlişki. *Sakarya Üniversitesi Eğitim Fakültesi Dergisi*, 0 (1).

21. Jalilian, F., Karami Matin, B., Ahmadpanah, M., Ataee, M., Ahmadi Jouybari, T., Eslami, A.A., Mirzaei Alavijeh, M. (2015). Socio-Demographic Characteristics Associated with Cigarettes Smoking, Drug Abuse and

Alcohol Drinking among Male Medical University Students in Iran. *J Res Health Sci.*; 15(1): 42–46.

22. Harding, J. F. (2015). Increases in Maternal Education and Low-Income Children's Cognitive and Behavioral Outcomes. *Developmental Psychology*, 51(5): 583–599.

23. Kuzlak, A., Çuvaş, B. & Sakallı-Uğurlu, N. (2017). Anne ve babaların eğitim düzeyi ve mesleki statüleri ile üniversite öğrencilerinin cinsiyetçilik ve muhafazakârlığı arasındaki ilişki. *Nesne*, 5(9): 89–109.

24. Cui, Y., Fan, R., Wang, Y. M., Kaye, A. J., Kaye, A. D., Bueno, F. R., & Pei, J. M. (2014). A Changing Healthcare System Model: The Effectiveness of Knowledge, Attitude, and Skill of Nursing Assistants Who Attend Senile Dementia Patients in Nursing Homes in Xi'an, China - A Questionnaire Survey. *The Ochsner Journal*, 14(3): 328–334.

25 .Ministry of Family and Social Policies. (2017). Türkiye'de Yaşlı Bakım Hizmetleri Raporu

Hayat Yalın and Necmiye Sabuncu

Handicap and Quality of Life of the Patients after Stroke

Abstract: Objective: Studying the validity and reliability of the London Handicap Scale (LHS), a general quality of life scale for patients with stroke, and to determine the functional status, disability and quality of life of people with stroke.

Material and Method: The study was carried out in two stages with volunteer patients whose ages ranged from 19 to 84 (mean 63.9 ± 13.9 years). In the first phase, the cultural adaptation and psychometric properties of the LHS were performed. In the second stage, functional status, handicap and quality of life of the patients with stroke were determined. Patient Information Form, LHS, Barthel Index (BI) and Modified Ranking Scale (mRS) were used for data collection. SPSS 17.0 program was used in the analysis and $p < 0.05$ was considered significant.

Results: Internal consistency coefficient determination, test-retest and parallel form methods were used in the scale reliability study. The internal consistency coefficient (Chronbach's alpha) was found as 0.901 for both the test and the retest. Scale validity, criterion-dependent validity and construct validity methods were used in the scale validity study. Correlation coefficients between BI and LHS were calculated as 0,837 for the test and 0,839 for retest. The factor load was found as 0.678–0.934 for the test and 0.701–0.941 for the retest. As a result of confirmatory factor analysis, the chi-square test result was found to be significant ($p = 0.043$). Since there was a high correlation between the scales used in the second part of the study ($r = 0.840$), it was found that the quality of life of the patients after stroke was directly related to their functional status and handicap.

Conclusion: As a result of this study; Turkish version of LHS was found to be a reliable and valid clinical tool for the assessment of handicap and quality of life of the patients after stroke.

Keywords: Stroke, Nursing care, Quality of life, London Handicap Scale

Introduction

Stroke is an important public health problem that causes high costs and death due to complications, disability and increased health expenditures (1, 2, 3).

Nursing care is important in the prevention of stroke disease and in both acute and later stages of the disease. Because of the negative changes that may occur in other systems of the body due to stroke, the development of complications with appropriate nursing interventions to be made in time can be prevented (4). The main objective of nursing care is to affect in a positive way the physical, social and psychological dimensions of the quality of life (5).

Physical and mental limitations and disability that develop after stroke adversely affect the individual's daily life activities and also limit the person's long-term care needs, health perception and social activities. Many patients who are bed-dependent because of stroke consider their condition as worse than death. Due to all these changes, the quality of life of the individual and the family is negatively affected (5,6).

The scales used for the evaluation of disability and quality of life of patients with stroke provide significant contributions about deficits caused by stroke, determination of functional and disability status of the patient, medical treatment, planning of nursing care and rehabilitation interventions, determination of change in neurological status, effectiveness of treatment, determination of discharge requirements and common language for healthcare team (7). For this reason, this study was carried out with the aim of determining validity and reliability studies of London Handicap Scale, which is a general quality of life scale, for patients who had a stroke in the Turkish population and then determining the functional status, disability and quality of life of the patients with stroke.

Material and Method

The research, which is planned as methodological and descriptive, consists of two parts. In the first part of the study, the cultural adaptation, validation and reliability studies of London Handicap Scale which was developed by Rowan H Harwood and Shah Ebrahim in England for chronic and progressive diseases were done. At this stage, patients who accepted to participate in the study were administered the Patient-Disease Identification Form which included sociodemographic characteristics and information about the disease, London Handicap Scale made of cultural adaptation (translation and language validity) and Barthel Index (BI). The application was carried out with two interviews. In the first interview, Patient-Disease Identification Form, the London Handicap Scale and Barthel Index were administered. In the second part of the study, in addition to the London Handicap Scale and Barthel Index (BI) the functional status, disability and quality of life of patients were determined by using the Modified Rankin Scale (mRS). The research was performed in general neurology and stroke outpatient clinics of an university hospital in İstanbul. The ethics committee approval of the study was obtained from the Research Ethics Committee of Marmara University Faculty of Medicine. Permission was obtained from the university hospital where the data was collected, and from those who developed the original scale. In addition, verbal and written information about the research was given to the patients who agreed to participate in the research and their names would be kept confidential. Their written informed consent was obtained.

Data Collection Tools

Data were collected by using the Patient-Disease Identification Form, London Handicap Scale, Barthel Index and Modified Rankin Scale.

Patient-Disease Identification Form was developed by the researcher using the current literature. The form consist of two parts as sociodemographic characteristics as age, educational and marital status, height, body weights, occupation, working status and disease identifications as stroke type, speech disorder and neurological deficit.

London Handicap Scale (LHS) is a general health-related quality of life scale developed by Harwood and Ebrahim in 1994 (8) in accordance with the criterias of International Classification of Impairments, Disabilities and Handicaps (ICIDH) that published by the World Health Organization (1993) (9). The scale consists of six parts (6 questions) and measures the health status of patients with chronic, proliferating, progressive diseases, including rehabilitation, and a disability profile (movement, physical independence, occupation, social relationship, adaptation and economic competence) and general disability severity in six different dimensions. Each question has six answer options (8). After the scale was developed, a scale validation study was performed by Jenkinson, Mant, Carter, Wade and Winner (10) in order to perform the scoring by using standard scoring system. They scored "5 points" for the best response options and "0 points" for the worst case, and found that the scale was valid with the standard scoring method. The high score obtained from the scale is interpreted as good quality of life. Filling the scale can be done by the patient or caregivers or the interviewer (8).

Barthel Index is a ten-item scale developed by Mahoney and Barthel in 1965 to evaluate physical independence in daily living activities as transfer, use of ambulation/wheelchair, climbing up and down stairs, feeding, dressing, taking care, bathing, toilet use, urinary incontinence, stool incontinence. Each item is scored on a three-point scoring system (between 0–15 points in 5-point increments according to the question) and the total score is calculated. The total score ranges from "0" to "100" which "0" are full addictions and "100" shows full independence (11).

Modified Rankin Scale (mRS) is a frequently used scale to determine the functional status of patients in the evaluation of the final condition of stroke.

This scale classifies the disability that develops after the stroke in six degrees, scoring between "0" and "5". The absence of any finding is scored as "0" and if there is serious disability or bed dependence, it is scored as "5". Having a mRS score of two or less is a good last condition, and being over two is defined as a bad last status marker.

The Universe and Sample of the Research

The universe of the study consisted of patients who had had previous stroke (ischemic or hemorrhagic) and had come to control during the study. In determining the sample number of the research the recommendation written in the literature as sample size in the scale studies should be 5–10 times of each scale item and was taken into consideration (12, 13, 14). For this reason, the sample of the study consisted of 30 patients who met the sample selection criteria for the first part of the study and 57 patients for the second part.

Sample selection criteria: In the study of Evans et al. (15) that was aimed to determine the quality of life of patients with stroke, patients were followed up for 3, 6 and 12 months after discharged from the hospital. As a result of this study, it was stated that the physical recovery in the patients was 3–6 months later and the need to climb the stairs provides personal hygiene and visiting their friends increased in time. Therefore, sample selection criteria were adult patients who had a stroke at least 3 months ago and who did not have any disability before the illness and who agreed to participate in the study.

Data analysis: The SPSS (Statistical Package for Social Sciences) for Windows 17.0 program was used to analyze the data (SPSS Inc. 2007) and the data were evaluated by a statistical expert. Kolmogorov-Smirnov distribution test was used for the evaluation of the normal distribution as well as descriptive statistical methods (Frequency, Percentage, Average, Standard deviation) while evaluating the study data. Mann Whitney U test was used for comparison of quantitative data, Kruskal Wallis test was used for the comparison of the groups which did not show normal distribution, and Spearman Correlation analysis was used to determine the relationships between the scales. The results were evaluated as 95 % confidence interval and $p < 0.05$ and $p < 0.01$, respectively.

LHS Validity Studies

Language validity, scope validity, construct validity and criterion validity methods were used in validity studies. The original scale was translated into Turkish by two independent researchers. The translations were brought together and the scale was created by selecting the most appropriate expressions. A presentation form was prepared for the expert opinion, which includes the Turkish articles of the scale and the Turkish equivalents of these items. The form was sent to experts to assess the compatibility and comprehensibility of the scale's English and Turkish equivalents. The experts were asked to indicate their recommendations in the form of each scale item. After the feedback received from the experts, necessary corrections were made and the final version of the scale was created. The final version of the scale was translated back into English. After the language validity of the scale, the Expert Opinion Presentation Form which was previously used in language validity studies was used to determine the content (scope) validity. The criterion validity was used in the validity study and the relationship between London Handicap Scale and Barthel Index was evaluated with Pearson correlation. Factor analysis was performed to determine the construct validity.

LHS Reliability Studies

Reliability is the assurance of invariance, competence, estimation, equivalence and consistency (16). Internal consistency analysis (Cronbach alpha), test-retest and parallel-form technique were used in the study.

The most commonly used method for examining internal consistency is Cronbach's Alpha Coefficient (17). In the literature, Cronbach's Alpha values greater than 0.50 are expected to be the limits for validation of the internal consistency of the scales, 0.70 and above for psychological tests and 0.80 and above for cognitive tests such as intelligence tests (17, 18, 19).

The test-retest technique is used to establish the reliability criterion for reliability. It is stated by experts that this period should be between two weeks and one month (16). Therefore, re-testing was applied to all participants within 2–4 weeks after the first test.

In parallel form reliability, also known as equivalent form reliability, an improved or adapted scale and its equivalent are applied to the same group. Correlation between the scale scores is calculated by the Pearson Product Moment formula, so the correlation between the two scales is examined (16). BI was used as a parallel form in the research for equivalent form reliability studies.

Determining Functional Status, Handicap and Quality of Life of Patients

After the cultural adaptation studies, the second part of the study was passed after the London Disability Scale was determined to be a reliable and valid tool for use in patients with stroke in the Turkish population. Functional status, disability and quality of life of patients were determined by using the Patient-Disease

Identification Form, London Handicap Scale, Barthel Index and Modified
Rankin Scale.

Results

The results obtained from the study are given in two main sections: the validity
of the London Handicap Scale for stroke patients and the functional status, disability and quality of life results of the patients after stroke.

Validity-Reliability Results

This section includes results about the scope validity, structure validity and reliability studies of the London Handicap Scale for patients with stroke. Expert
opinions were used to determine the scope validity. Scope validity studies and
scope validity index values were obtained by using both Lawshe technique and
Davis technique and compared with Lawshe's Minimum Scope Validity Rates
Table (20). Because the calculated values were higher than the minimum value
in the table, it was decided that there was agreement between the experts. Scope
validity index was calculated as 98 % across the scale. The internal consistency
value of the London Handicap Scale (Cronbach alpha) was 0.901 for test and
0.901 for re-test. When the item's total correlations are examined with respect
to internal consistency level and scale questions, for the test, it ranged from
0.577 to 0.900, and in the range of 0.600 to 0.903 for retest (Tab. 1). The internal

Tab. 1: London Handicap Scale Structure Validity and Reliability Results

Questions	Test		Retest	
	Factor Load	Item-Total Correlation	Factor Load	Item-Total Correlation
Does your health stop you from getting around?	0,877	0,821	0,852	0,788
Does your health stop you looking after yourself?	0,934	0,900	0,926	0,891
Does your health limit your work or leisure activities?	0,917	0,862	0,941	0,903
Does your health stop you getting on with people?	0,771	0,676	0,746	0,647
Does your health stop you understanding the world around you?	0,678	0,577	0,701	0,600
Are you able to afford the things you need?	0,759	0,674	0,770	0,684

consistency of the London Handicap Scale was established. There was no significant difference in terms of questions and total scale scores (p> 0.05) (Tab. 2) between the test-retest averages of the LHS; The correlation coefficients obtained by the test-retest method of the LHS ranged from r=0,946 to r=0,999 (p <0,001). In this framework, the results of the test showed that the results were stable in every application of the scale.

As a result of the factor analysis performed to determine the construct validity of the scale, a single factor (single structure = disability) was observed. Factor loads for testing ranged from 0.678 to 0.934; for retesting, it ranged from 0.701 to 0.941 (Tab. 2). Factor analysis of the London Handicap Scale test-retest factor was found to be considerably high. The Barthel Index was used as a parallel test for the quality-f-life questionnaire, which is frequently used in stroke patients and questioning daily life activities. The correlation coefficient obtained by the test-parallel test method of the London Handicap Scale was r = 0,837 and the correlation coefficient obtained by the retest-parallel test method was r = 0,839 (p <0,001). In this context, the test results show that London Handicap Scale gives stable results based on the Barthel Index scale.

Results of Patients' Handicap, Functional Status and Quality of Life after Stroke

This part of the study was performed on 57 patients that living in Turkey and who have spent at least three months after stroke, ranging in age from 19 to 84 and 31 (54.4 %) were male. The mean age of all patients was 63.9 ± 13.9 years. Twenty-four (38.6 %) patients were in the age group of 71 and over, 30 (52.6 %)

Tab. 2: London Handicap Scale Test and Retest Results

	Test		Retest		
Questions	**Mean**	**SD**	**Mean**	**SD**	**p**
Does your health stop you from getting around?	3,50	1,14	3,50	1,11	0,999
Does your health stop you looking after yourself?	3,10	1,52	3,20	1,45	0,184
Does your health limit your work or leisure activities?	2,90	1,45	3,00	1,51	0,184
Does your health stop you getting on with people?	4,30	0,79	4,33	0,80	0,326
Does your health stop you understanding the world around you?	4,00	0,71	4,00	0,71	-
Are you able to afford the things you need?	3,97	1,03	4,03	1,03	0,161
London Handicap Scale Score	**74,77**	**18,75**	**75,78**	**18,67**	**0,083**

were overweight, 14 (24.6 %) were Class I obese, 41 were (71.9 %) married and 19 (33.3 %) were in primary education. All of the participants have social security. In addition, 21 (36.8 %) were housewives and one (1.8 %) was student, only 3 (5.3 %) of them work actively (Tab. 3).

Most of all cases (33.3 %; n = 19) were found to have stroke 13–36 months ago. Stroke type was ischemia at 52 (91.2 %) patients and 18 patients (34.6 %) had LACI (Lakuner Infarcts). Eight (14.0 %) of them had mild–moderate aphasia and 14 (24.6 %) had motor and sensory loss (deficits) on the right side both lower and upper extremities. All of the cases obeyed orders and had place orientations (Tab. 4).

The mean total score of the London Handicap Scale was 76.7, and the average score of the orientation sub-dimension (item) was 4.7 points, and the average score of job, occupation and occupancy dimension was found to be the lowest with 3.2. Values determined for Barthel Index as 86,40 ± 17,23 (30–100) and for mRS as 1.80 ± 1.35 (0–4) (Tab. 5).

London Handicap Scale, Barthel Index and mRS scores did not show any significant change according to gender, age groups, body mass index, marital status, educational status and occupations (p> 0.05). However, it was found that the scale scores showed a significant change according to the study status of the cases (p <0.05). All three scale scores of the subjects did not show a significant change according to the type of stroke, clinical and etiological classification of ischemic stroke (p> 0.05).

London Handicap Scale scores (53,33 ± 9,76) and Barthel Index Scores (62,5 ± 9,64) in patients with mild-to-moderate aphasia, and scores of patients with normal speech status (LHS score 80,54 ± 16 BI score 90,10 ± 15,12) were significantly lower and modified Rankin Scale score (3,37 ± 0,52) was significantly higher (1,57 ± 1,28) (p <0,01) (Tab. 6).

Modified Rankin Scale score was found to be significantly higher in patients with deficits in the right arm (2.43 ± 1.38) than in those without (1,61±1,38) (P <0.05). The patients' LHS score and BI scores did not show a significant change according to the deficit status in the right arm (p> 0.05). Subjects with deficit in the left arm had lower scores from both LHS (62,91 ± 7,49) and BI (74,06 ± 13,93) than those without (P <0.01). The patients with deficits in the left arm had significantly higher scores than those without mRS score (2,94 ± 0,93) (1,37 ± 1,22) (p <0,01). The patients' LHS and BI scores did not show a significant change (p> 0,05) in the right leg compared to the presence of deficits in the right leg, but the score of the mRS score (2,43 ± 1,02) was not significant (1,61 ± 1,38). It was found to be significantly higher (p <0.05). The LHS (61,76 ± 8,67) and BI

Tab. 3: Distribution of Descriptive Characteristics

		Female		Male		Total	
		n	%	n	%	n	%
Age	Under 50	6	23,1	6	19,4	12	21,1
	51–60	7	26,9	4	12,9	11	19,3
	61–70	5	19,2	7	22,6	12	21,1
	Over 71	8	30,8	14	45,2	22	38,6
Body Mass Index (BMI)	Normal	3	11,5	10	32,3	13	22,8
	Overweight	13	50,0	17	54,8	30	52,6
	Class I Obesity	10	38,5	4	12,9	14	24,6
Marital status	Married	13	50,0	28	90,3	41	71,9
	Single	13	50,0	3	9,7	16	28,1
Education level	Illiterate	2	7,7	0	0,0	2	3,5
	Literate	7	26,9	1	3,2	8	14,0
	Primary school	11	42,3	8	25,8	19	33,3
	Middle School	3	11,5	6	19,4	9	15,8
	High school	3	11,5	8	25,8	11	19,3
	University	0	0,0	6	19,4	6	10,5
	Postgraduate	0	0,0	2	6,5	2	3,5
Profession	Technical employee (electrician, civil engineer)	0	0,0	2	6,5	2	3,5
	Trade and self-employment	1	3,8	8	25,8	9	15,8
	Public employees (faculty member, officer, teacher, prosecutor)	1	3,8	10	32,3	11	19,3
	Manager	0	0	5	16,1	5	8,8
	Worker	2	7,7	6	19,4	8	14,0
	Other	21	80,8	0	0,0	21	36,8
	housewife student	1	3,8	0	0,0	1	1,8
Working status	Yes	0	0,0	3	9,7	3	5,3
	No	26	100,0	28	90,3	54	94,7
The reason for not working	Housewife	21	80,8	0	0,0	21	38,9
	Retired	3	11,5	27	96,4	30	55,6
	Other (due to student, illness)	2	7,7	1	3,6	3	5,6 %
Having social security	Yes	26	100,0	31	100,0	57	100,0

Tab. 4: Distribution of the Signs and Complications of the Stroke

		n	%
Stroke type	Hemorrhage	5	8,8
	Ischemia	52	91,2
Localization of Hemorrhagic Stroke	Lober	4	80,0
	Subcortical	1	20,0
Ischemic Stroke Clinical Classification	TACI	7	13,5
	PACI	16	30,8
	LACI	18	34,6
	POCI	11	21,2
Ischemic Stroke Etiology Classification	Wide artery atherothrombosis	12	23,1
	Cardioembolizm	8	15,4
	Small vessel occlusion	28	53,8
	Rare etiology	2	3,8
	Unspecified etiology	2	3,8
Time to pass the disease	3-6 months	9	15,8
	6-12 months	16	28,1
	13-36 months	19	33,3
	Over 37 months	13	22,8
Speeking	Normal	49	86,0
	Light-Medium Aphasia	8	14,0
Deficit in the right arm	No	43	75,4
	Yes	14	24,6
Deficit in the left arm	No	41	71,9
	Yes	16	28,1
Deficit in the right leg	No	43	75,4
	Yes	14	24,6
Deficit in the left leg	No	40	70,2
	Yes	17	29,8
Compliance with Orders	Yes	57	100
Place Orientation	Yes	57	100

scores (71,47 ± 17,21) were significantly lower and mRS scores were significantly higher (3.00 ± 0.94) of the patients with a deficit in the left leg (p <0.01).

Discussion

The results obtained from the cultural adaptation of LHS and functional status, disability and quality of life of individuals with stroke were discussed under two

Tab. 5: Distribution of Total and Item Scores of London Handicap Scale

	Mean	SD	Median	IQR	Min - Max
Total LHS Score	76,7	18,1	80	31,7	40 - 100
Mobility	3,6	1,2	4,0	2,0	0 - 5
Physical independence	3,5	1,5	4,0	3,0	0 - 5
Work, occupation	3,2	1,5	3,0	2,5	0 - 5
Social integration	4,3	0,8	4,0	1,0	2 - 5
Orientation	4,7	0,7	5,0	0,0	2 - 5
Economic competence	3,7	1,0	4,0	2,0	1 - 5

Tab. 6: Comparison of Scale Scores by Speech Status of Cases

Scale	Speech Status	n	Mean	SD	p
LHS Score	Normal	49	80,541	16,164	0,000**
	Light-Medium Aphasia	8	53,330	9,758	
mRS Score	Normal	49	1,551	1,259	0,000**
	Light-Medium Aphasia	8	3,375	0,518	
BI Score	Normal	49	90,204	15,033	0,000**
	Light-Medium Aphasia	8	63,125	10,329	

** $p < 0,01$

headings as cultural adaptation of london handicap scale and functional status, disability and quality of life of patients after stroke.

Cultural Adaptation of the London Handicap Scale

Stroke is the most common neurological disorder in the world (1). The physical and mental limitations, handicap, pain and depression that develop after stroke adversely affect the individual's daily life activities and also limit the person's long-term care needs, health perception and social activities (5). To determine the health-related quality of life of the patients after stroke, many scales have been developed for both general and special purposes (21, 22, 23, 24). One of these scales is the London Handicap Scale (LHS), which was developed in the United Kingdom (UK) to determine the effects of disability and handicap on patients' quality of life in chronic, progressive and multiple diseases (8, 25). Cultural adaptation of LHS was done in many different countries such as Hong Kong, Sweden, Netherlands and Nigeria (26, 27, 28).

Cultural adaptation of scales is as important as developing a new scale. The scales that have not been culturally adapted, no matter how well translated, cannot serve the purpose. Cultural adaptation studies are carried out in two stages, namely the translation of the scale from the original language into the target language and the evaluation of the scale with psychometric tests (29).

Translation

The basic prerequisite adopted in scale translation is conceptual equivalence. Translation studies are recommended to take place in three stages as advanced translation, back translation and pre-implementation (29). The London Handicap Scale, which is in English, has been translated into Turkish by two independent individuals. For the language validity study of the scale, Expert Opinion form which consisted both English and Turkish items of scale was used and sent to 10 experts. After the feedback received from the experts, necessary corrections were made and the final version of the scale was created. The final version of the scale was translated back into English.

In the cultural adaptation studies of the London Handicap Scale in Sweden, advanced translation was carried out by three different people in the past. The first translator translated the scale from English to Swedish. The second person checked the first translation and made minor changes, and the third person checked the fluency of the content (30). In the case of Nigeria, the translation was done by 3 different translators working in the university, using the reverse-back translation technique. In the translation, it was determined that the orientation and economic competence sub-dimensions of the scale were not suitable and necessary corrections were made (28). There is no information on scale translation in articles including Hong Kong and Dutch adaptation studies (26, 27).

Psychometric Tests

The scale was first translated from the original language into the target language. The final version was applied to 30 patients and language and content (scope) validity, construct validity and reliability were tested. Scope validity is to determine the extent to which the scale and each item of the scale serve the purpose as a whole. Scope validity rates were developed by Lawshe (1975). After the language validity of the scale, the Expert Opinion Presentation Form which was used in the language validity studies was used to determine the content validity. The scope validity ratio and scope validity index results of the London Handicap

Scale were compared with the Lawshe's Minimum Scope Validity table (31). The scope validity index of the questions was determined as 80 %. There was no statistically significant difference between the scores given by the experts to the scale items in terms of both the general explanation (Kendall's W = 0.120, p = 0.306) and the question (Kendall 0,1s W = 0.111, p = 0.310).

Internal consistency analysis (Cronbach alpha) and test-retest technique were used for reliability analysis of the scale. The internal consistency value of the London Handicap Scale (Cronbachs alpha) with a total of 6 questions was calculated as 0.901; The internal consistency value of the retest (Cronbach's alpha) was found as 0.901. Test-retest reliability levels were equal and at this level, and the internal consistency of the LHS was found to be quite high. Harwood et al. (8) found that the reliability coefficient was 0.91 in patients with stroke and 0.70–0.80 in the Swedish version of the scale (30) and in Park and Choi (32) these values were 0.85. Jenkinson et al. (10) in their study have determined the validity of LHS scoring by standard scoring method and in these studies the scale Cronbach alpha value was 0.98. Our results are similar to those of Harwood et al. and Jankinson et al. The results are higher than the results of Westergren and Hagel, which regulate the Swedish version, and Park and Choi.

In the test-retest method (after 2–4 weeks after the first test), the data were collected by face-to-face interviews with the patients. Differences between the means for the Test-Retest Scale of LHS was examined. There was no significant difference in terms of questions and total scale scores. It was found that the correlation coefficients ranged from r = 0,86 to r = 0,97. The item-total correlations of the London Handicap Scale were obtained for testing (0.577–0.900) – for retesting (0.600–0.903) and were found to be high at acceptable levels.

Structure validity is a method that numerically reveals whether the items within the scale measure a single concept or several concepts when considered as a whole. Factor analysis is used to determine the construct validity of the scales (19). As a result of the factor analysis conducted to determine the construct validity of the scale, the factor loads changed between 0,678 and 0,934 for testing and between 0,701 and 0,941 for retest. Factor analysis of factor – test for re-test was found to be acceptable.

In the study, the correlation coefficient obtained by the parallel test method of London Handicap Scale was r = 0,837 for the test and r = 0,839 for the re-test. In this context, the test results show that London Handicap Scale gives stable results based on the Barthel Scale. It is reported that there is a high level of correlation between LHS and BI in both the original scale (8) and the cultural adaptation study in Sweden (10).

Functional Status, Handicap and Quality of Life of Patients

The mean scores of the subjects were 76.72 ± 18.08 (40–100) for London Handicap Scale, 1.80 ± 1.35 (0–4) for modified Rankin Scale and 86.40 ± 17,23 (30–100) for Barthel Index. In the study of Gall et al. (33) the mean score of LHS was determined as 73.

The Mean score of BI was reported as 95,5 (SD = 8,9) by Muus et al. (34), 50,85 ± 22,27 by Gündüz and Erhan (35) and 17.62 (0–20) by Pan et al. (36). Pan at al (36) also reported the mean score of LHS as 14.63 (range 6–31). Sturm et al. (37) found that the mean score of LHS was 72.

The mean subscale scores of the London Handicap Scale were 3.6 for mobility, 3.5 for physical independence, 3.2 for occupation, 4.3 for social integration, 4.7 for orientation and 3.7 for economic qualification. Sturm et al. (37) determined that patients with stroke experienced wider handicap when the physical independence and orientation sub-dimensions of the BI were severely affected. At the same time, they stated that the inadequacy and handicap, which will decrease after acute stroke treatment, will have an effect on handicap development. Correlation analysis of all three scales was performed and a significant correlation was found between the scales as 82 % and 88.1 %. Thus, it was concluded that all three scales had a high level of coherence and similar results.

The study was performed on a total of 57 patients aged between 19 and 84 years with stroke and at least three months prior to stroke. The mean age of all patients was 63.9 ± 13.9 years. London Handicap Scale, Modified Rankin Scale and Barthel Index scores did not show a significant change (p> 0.05), but the scores of patients aged 61 and over were lower than those of younger patients. In a study conducted by Gündüz and Erhan (35), it was stated that there was no significant relationship between BI and age. In some studies, it is stated that advanced age affects the quality of life of stroke patients negatively. Sharma et al. (38) reported that the quality of life of patients aged 75 years and older was lower. Among the causes of these contradictions between advanced age and quality of life, diabetes, hypertension and cardiac diseases with increased incidence and the loss of function caused by these diseases can be counted. Therefore, it is accepted that age alone does not have an effect on the quality of life of stroke patients (39).

Scores of LHS, mRS and BI did not change significantly by gender (p> 0.05). However, the mean score of the females and the mean score of the mRS were worse than the males, but the mean BI score was found to be approximately the same. Gray et al. (40) in the study performed by women in the mRS mean score and the BI average score is worse than that of men. Sturm et al. (41, 42) found that the post-stroke quality of life was significantly lower in female patients than in male patients. In the studies performed by Şenocak et al. (43), there was no difference between the gender in terms of quality of life.

Body mass index was found to be normal in 22.8 % of patients, 52.6 % were overweight and 24.6 % were in Class I obesity. The rate of obesity (38.5 %) was significantly higher in female cases (p <0.05). The scores obtained from all scales did not show a significant difference according to body mass index (p> 0.05), but the mean scores of all three scales in the body mass index were better than those in the other group. It is known that obesity, which is one of the most important health problems of today, causes many diseases from heart diseases to cancer.

Most of the cases (71.9 %) were married. The rate of being married (90.3 %) in male cases was significantly higher than female (50 %) (p <0.01). However, no significant change was observed when the scale scores and marital status were compared (p> 0.05). In some studies, although marital status (being married) is stated to be one of the main determinants of quality of life in patients with stroke (44, 45), a significant relationship between BI value and marital status could not be found in a study conducted by Gündüz and Erhan (35).

It was found that the scores of the subjects did not show a significant change according to their educational status (p> 0.05), but the scale scores improved in parallel with the increasing level of education. When the study status of the cases was questioned, it was learned that 94.7 % did not work. 36.8 % of the cases who did not work were housewives, 52.6 % were retired and 5.3 % were not working due to student or illness. All of the cases were found to have social security. In the studies performed, the return to work in stroke patients was reported as one of the main determinants of quality of life (46). In this study, it was found that the London Handicap Scale score of the patients showed a significant change according to their study status (p <0.05). LHS score (96,66 ± 3,33) was significantly higher in the study group than in the non-working cases (75,61 ± 17,92). Thus, it was found that the quality of life of the employees was better than those who did not work.

The rate of stroke in patients was 8,8 % hemorrhage (80 % lobar, 20 % subcortical) and 91,2 % ischemia. In the literature it is stated that approximately 15–20 % of all strokes in the world are caused by hemorrhage and 80–85 % is caused by ischemia (47, 48). In different studies conducted in our country have been reported 66.3 % (49), 95.9 % (50) and 77 % (51) of the patients had ischemic stroke. Lo et al. (52) reported that 93.1 % of cases had ischemic stroke in a study conducted in China. Stroke type compared with scale scores and it was found that the scores of all three scales did not show a significant change according to the type of stroke (p> 0.05). Owolabi (53) stated that the study did not have a significant effect on the quality of life of the stroke type.

In the clinical classification of patients with ischemic stroke, 13.5 % had TACI (Total Anterior Circulation Infarcts), 30.8 % had PACI (Partial Anterior Circulation Infarcts), 34.6 % had LACI (Lacunar Infarcts) and 21,2 % were POCI (Posterior Circulation Infarcts). In the etiological classification distribution of stroke patients, 23.1 % had large artery atherothrombosis, 15.4 % had cardioembolism, 53.8 % had small vessel occlusion, 3.8 % had rare etiology and 3.8 % had not been classified. In the literature, TOAST with ischemic stroke etiology and its incidence are defined as large/large arterial atherosclerosis (thrombosis or embolism) 20 %, cardioembolism 20 %, small vessel occlusion (lacun) 25 %, other etiologic causes 5 % and unexplained 30 % (54). The scale scores of the patients with stroke type ischemia were not significantly different according to the clinical and etiological classification of ischemic stroke (p> 0.05). However, the lowest scores in all three scales were found to belong to PACI ischemic stroke clinical class. Sturn et al. (37, 42) reported that both the LHS and BI scores of patients with TACI ischemic stroke were worse than others.

When the time to pass the disease was questioned, it was found that 15.8 % of the cases had stroke 3–6 months ago, 28.1 % of cases were 6–12 months, 33.3 % were 1–3 years and 22.8 % were 4 years and before. In the study performed by Gündüz and Erhan (35), the mean time of stroke was 14 ± 10.7 months (range 7–40 months).

In this study, it was determined that 86 % of the cases had normal speech status and 14 % had mild-moderate aphasia. Muus et al. (34) reported that 35 % of the patients had speech disorder. When the motor and sensory loss (deficits) in the extremities of the patients were investigated, there were no deficits in 43.86 % of the cases.Deficits in the extremities were found in 24.56 % of the cases with 22.18% involving the left arm and leg, and 22.18 % involving the right arm and leg. Motor and/or sensory losses were detected only in the left arm in 1.75% of the cases,only in the left leg in 5.26 % of the cases, and only in the right leg in 1.75 %of the cases. In the LHS adaptation study in Nigeria, 60 % of patients were affected by the right sides of their bodies (28). In the study, it was found that the cases with deficits in the right arm and right leg had significantly higher (p <0.05) than the patients without mRS score and no significant change in LHS score and BI scores (p> 0.05). The scores of patients with deficits in the left arm were significantly lower than those without LHS score and the score of subjects without BI score (p <0.01), and they were significantly higher than those without mRS score (p <0.01). The same result was found in cases with deficits in the left leg. Şenocak et al. (43) compared the quality of life of patients with right and left side stroke and no significant difference was found.

In some studies, quality of life scores were reported to be worse in patients with right hemiparesis than those with left hemiparesis (39). In our study, this result, which was determined differently from the literature, could not be evaluated exactly because the patients used their hands predominantly. However, we think that the hand, which is not normally used, shows how effective it is in our daily functions.

Conclusion

As a result, it was determined that London Handicap Scale is a valid and reliable scale that can be used to determine the handicap severity and quality of life of patients after stroke in our country. Some of the proposed studies related to the scale in the future due to the ease of implementation are listed below.

1. Evaluation of patients who are not only in outpatients clinics but also patients with high dependence on beds and care,
2. Evaluation handicap and quality of life of the patients at certain time intervals after stroke (3 months, 6 months and 1 year etc.),
3. Psychometric measurements of the scale for people with different chronic diseases such as multiple sclerosis, rheumatoid arthritis, etc.
4. Psychometric measurements of the scale for people with disability such as leg amputation etc.

Limitations of the Study

The study was conducted in a hospital. It was also observed that many of the patients who volunteered to participate in the research were coming to the hospital on their own. Patients who were more severe or had a higher level of physical dependence were not observed in the outpatients clinic due to the inadequacy of current conditions, difficulties in mobilization and transport of patients.

Financial Disclosure

The authors declared that they did not receive financial support for this study.

The results of the validity and reliability of the first part of the study were presented as a poster presentation at the 15th International Nursing Research Conference and the second part as a poster presentation at The 1st International Clinical Nursing Research Congress.

References

1. Sacco R (2008). Serebrovasküler Hastalığın Patogenezi, Sınıflandırılması ve Epidemiyolojisi. İçinde: *Türkçe Merrit's Neurology*, Ed Rowland LP, Çev Ed: Baslo B, Gürses C. 11. Baskı, Güneş Tıp Kitabevleri, Ankara, 275–290.

2. Yatsu, F. (2008). İnmenin Tedavisi ve Önlenmesi. İçinde Merritt's Türkçe Neurology. Ed. Rowland L., Çev. ed. Baslo B., Gürses C., Güneş Tıp Kitabevleri, Ankara, 324.

3. Kalra L. (2009). Medical Complications of Stroke. In: *Stroke Recovery and Rehabilitation*. Eds: Stein J, Harvey RL, Macko RF, Winstein CJ, Zorowitz RD, Demos Medical Publishing, USA, p. 405–412.

4. Karadakovan A. (2010). Sinir Sistemi Hastalıkları. İçinde: Dahili ve Cerrahi Hastalıklarda Bakım, Ed. Karadakovan A., Aslan FE., Nobel Kitabevi, Adana, 1176–1195.

5. Akdemir N. (2003). Hemşirelik Uygulamalarında Temel Kavramlar. Ed. Akdemir N, Birol L, İç Hastalıları ve Hemşirelik Bakımı. 1. Baskı. Vehbi Koç Vakfı SANERC Yayınları, No: 2, Istanbul, 3–24.

6. Özdemir G. (2000). Beyin Krizi Nedir? Hakkında Bilmek İstedikleriniz. *Eskişehir Türk Beyin Damar Hastalıkları Derneği Yayınları* No: 3: 5–27.

7. Anderson P, Lloyd A. (2001). Outcomes Research and Health Economics. In: *Principles of Clinical Researh*. Ed. Giovanna I., Hayes G.Wrıghston Bıomedical Publishing Ltd, Philadelphia.

8. Harwood RH, Gompertz P, Ebrahim S (1994). Handicap One Year after a Stroke: Validity of a New Scale. *J Neurol Neurosurg Psychiatry*; 57: 825–829.

9. World Health Organization (2001). *International Classification of Functioning, Disability, and Health*. Geneva, Switzerland..

10. Jenkinson C, Mant J, Carter J, Wade D, Winner S. (2000). The London Handicap Scale: A Re-Evalution of Its Validity Using Standard Scoring and Summation. *J Neurol Neurosurg Psychiatry*; 68; 365–367.

11. Mahoney FI, Barthel DW. (1965). Functional Evaluation: The Barthel Index. *Maryland State Med J*, 14:61–65.

12. Çimen S., Bahar Z., Öztürk C., Bektaş M. (2005) AIDS tutum ölçeğinin geçerlik ve güvenirlik çalışması. *Zonguldak Sağlık Yüksekokulu Sağlık Eğitim Araştırma Dergisi*, 1: 111.

13. Ergül Ş., Bayık Temel A. (2007). Maneviyat ve manevi bakım dereceleme ölçeğinin Türkçe formunun geçerlik ve güvenirliği. Ege Üniversitesi Hemşirelik Yüksekokulu Dergisi, 23 (1): 75–87.

14. Tavşancıl E. (2006). Tutumların Ölçülmesi ve SPSS ile Veri Analizi, Nobel Yayın Dağıtım, Ankara.

15. Evans RL, Bishop DS, Matlock AL, Stranahan S, Noonan C (1987). Predicting Poststroke Family Function: A Continuing Dilemma, *Psychol Rep*, 60: 691–695.

16. Gözüm S, Aksayan S. (2003). Kültürler arası ölçek uyarlaması için rehber II: psikometrik özellikler ve kültürlerarası karşılaştırma, *Hemşirelikte Araştırma Geliştirme Dergisi*, 5(1): 9–14.

17. Şencan H. (2005). Sosyal ve Davranışsal Ölçümlerde Güvenilirlik ve Geçerlilik. 1. Baskı, Seçkin Yayınevi, Ankara.

18. Erefe İ (2002) (Ed.). Veri Toplama Araçlarının Niteliği. Hemşirelikte Araştırma İlke Süreç ve Yöntemleri. Odak Ofset, Ankara, 169–188.

19. Büyüköztürk Ş. (2009). Sosyal Bilimler İçin Veri Analizi El Kitabı. 10.Baskı, Pegem Akademi Yayıncılık, Ankara.

20. Lawshe, C.H. (1975). A Quantıtatıve Approach to Content Validity, *Personnel Psychology*, 28: 563–575.

21. Linden PD, Hanston L. (1998). Assesment Scales Fort the Evaluation of Stroke Patients. *J Stroke Cerebrovasc Dis*; 7(2): 113–127.

22. Couldhard-Morris, L. (2000). Clinical and Rehabilitation Outcome Measures. In Multiple Sclerosis: Diagnosis, Medical Management and Rehabilitation. Eds. Burks JS, Johnson KP. Demos Medical Publishing Inc, USA.

23. Kasney SE: (2006). Clinical Interpretation and Use of Stroke Scales. *The Lancet Neurology*, 5(7): 603–612.

24. Eyigör S. (2007). İnmeli hastada rehabilitasyon prensipleri. *Türk Fiz Tıp Rehab Derg*; 53(1): 19–25.

25. Harwood RH, Ebrahim S (1995). *Manual of the London Handicap Scale. Nothingam Department of Health Care of the Elderly*, University of Nothingam.

26. Lo RSK, Harwood R, Woo J, Yeung F, Ebrahim S (2001). Cross-Cultural Validation of the London Handicap Scale in Hong Kong Chinese. *Clin Rehabil.*, 15: 177–185.

27. Groothuis-Oudshoorn, CGM; Chorus AMJ, Beekum WT, Detmar SB, Hout WB. (2006). Modelling and Estimation of Valuations Fort the Dutch London Handicap Scale. *Journal of Health Economics*, 25:6, 119–1138.

28. 61- HT, Oluwatitofunmi PG: (2009). The London Handicap Scale: Validation of a Yoruba (Nigerian) Version among Stroke Survivors. *African Jeurnal of Neurological Sciences*; 28:1. 61–66.

29. Eser E.(2004). Sağlıkta Yaşam Kalitesi (SYK) Kavramı: Bir giriş denemesi, 1. Sağlıkta Yaşam Kalitesi Sempozyumu, İzmir.

30. Westergren A, Hagel P. (2006). Initial Validation of the Swedish Version of the London Handicap Scale. *Quality of Life Research*; 15: 1251–1256.

31. Özdamar K. (2004). Paket Programları ile İstatistiksel Veri Analizi-2 (Çok Değişkenli Analizler), Cilt 2, 4. Baskı, Kaan Kitabevi, Eskişehir, s. 235–276.

32. Park EY, Choi YI (2014). Rasch 1-7. Analysis of the London Handicap Scale in Stroke Patients: A Cross-Sectional Study, *J Neuroeng Rehabil*, 11: 114.

33. Gall SL, Dewey HM, Sturm JW, Macdonell RA, Thrift AG (2009). Handicap 5 Years After Stroke in the North East Melbourne Stroke Incidence Study. *Cerebrovasculer Dis J*, 27 (2):123–130.

34. Muus I, Petzold M, Ringsberg KC. (2009). Health-Related Quality of Life After Stroke: Reliability of Proxy Responses, *Clinical Nursing Research*, 18; 103–118.

35. Gündüz B, Erhan B. (2008). Quality of Life of Stroke Patients' Spouses Living in the Community in Turkey: Controlled Study with Short Form-36 Questionnaire. *Journal of Neurological Sciences* (Turkish) 25: (4) 17; 226–234.

36. Pan JH, Song XY, Lee SY, Kwok T. (2008). Longitudinal Analysis of Quality of Life for Stroke Survivors Using latent Curve Models, *Stroke*, 39: 2795–2802.

37. Sturm JW, Dewey HM., Donnan GA., Macdonell RAL., McNeil JJ., Thrift AG. (2002). Handicap after Stroke: How Does It Relate to Disability, Perception of Recovery, and Stroke Subtype?: The North East Melbourne Stroke Incidence Study (NEMESIS). *Stroke*, 33: 762–768.

38. Sharma JC, Fletcher S, Vassallo M. (1999) Strokes in the Elderly – Higher Acute and 3-Month Mortality – an Explanation. *Cerebrovasc Dis*, 9: 2–9.

39. Durmaz B., Atamaz F. (2006). İnme ve Hayat Kalitesi. *Fiziksel Tıp ve Rehabilitasyon Dergisi*; 52 özel ek B: B45–B49

40. Gray LJ, Sprigg N, Bath PMW, Boysen G, Deyn PPD, Leys D, ONeill D, Ringelstein EB, TAIST Investigators (2007). Sex Differences in Quality of Life in Stroke Survivors. Data From the Tinzaparin in Acute Ischaemic Stroke Trial (TAIST), *Stroke*. 38(11):2960-4.

41. Sturm JW, Osborne RH, Dewey HM, Donnan GA, Macdonell RAL, Thrift AG. (2002). Brief Comprehensive Quality of Life Assesment After Stroke: The Assesment of Quality of Life Instrument in the North East Melbourne Stroke Incidence Study (NEMESIS). *Stroke*, 33: 2888–2894.

42. Sturm JW, Donnan GA, Dewey HM, Macdonell RAL, Gilligan AK, Srikanth V, Thrift AG. (2004). Quality of Life After Stroke. The North East Melbourne Stroke Incidence Study (NEMESIS). Stroke, 35: 2340–2345.

43. Şenocak Ö, El G, Söylev GÖ, Avcılar S, Peker Ö. (2008). İnme Sonrasında Yaşam Kalitesini Etkileyen Faktörler. *Journal of Neurological Sciences (Turkish)* 25(3): 15; 169–175.

44. Bethoux F, Calmels P, Gautheron V. (1999). Changes in the Quality of Life of Hemiplegic Stroke Patients with Time. *Am J Phys Med Rehabil*, 78:19–23.

45. Kim P, Warren S, Madill H, Hadley M. (1999). Quality of Life of Stroke Survivors. *Qual Life Res*, 8: 293–301.

46. Küçükdeveci AA (2005). Rehabilitasyonda Yaşam Kalitesi. *Türk Fiz Tıp Derg*, 51 (Özel Ek B):B23–B29.

47. Bakar M, Oğul E. (2009). Tıkayıcı tip Beyin Damar Hastalıkları. İçinde: *Serebrovasküler Hastalıklar*, Ed Balkan S, 3. Baskı, Güneş Tıp Kitabevleri, Ankara, 71–74.

48. Can U. (2009). Hemorajik İnfarktlar. İçinde: *Serebrovasküler Hastalıklar*, Ed Balkan S, 3. Baskı, Güneş Tıp Kitabevleri, Ankara, 109–122.

49. Eskiyurt N, Yalıman A, Vural M, Kızıltaş H, Bölükbaş N, Çeşme F. (2005). İnmeli Olguların Özellikleri ve Fonksiyonel Durum Sonuçları. *İstanbul Tıp Fakültesi Dergisi*, 68:71–77.

50. Benbir G, Gözükırmızı E. (2007). Akut Serebrovasküler Hastalık Sonrası Erken Dönemde Depresyon. *Yeni Seymposium Journal*, 44 (1): 44–48.

51. Kumral E. (2009). Serebrovasküler Hastalıkların Epidemiyolojisi. İçinde: *Serebrovasküler Hastalıklar*, Ed Balkan S, 3. Baskı, Güneş Tıp Kitabevleri, Ankara, 37–50.

52 .Lo RSK, Cheng JOY, Wong EMC, Tang WK, Wong LKS,Woo J, Kwok T. (2008). Handicap and Its Determinants of Change in Stroke Survivorrs: One-Year Follow-up Study, *Stroke*, 39: 148–153.

53. Owolabi M.O. (2010): What Are the Consistent Predictors of Generic and Specific Post- stSroke Health-Related Quality of Life? *Cerebrovasc Dis*. 29(2), 105–10.

54. Warlow CP, Dennis MS, Gijn J, Hankey GJ, Sandercock PAG, Bamford JM, Wardlaw JM. (2001). *Stroke: APractical Guide to Management*. 2nd edition, Blackwell Science Ltd, USA.

Fadime Çınar, Fatma Eti Aslan, and Hayat Yalın

An Investigation of X and Y Generation Nurses Ethical Values

Abstract: Objective: In addition to medical practices and treatment process, nursing care and compliance of nurses with ethical values are of vital importance for health. For this reason, nursing practices and ethics have been mentioned in many studies. On the other hand, there are not enough studies on the effect of changing generations and their common characteristics on the ethical values of nurses. Therefore, it was aimed to investigate the difference between the levels of susceptibility of nurses in different generations to ethical values.

Material and Method: In this descriptive and cross-sectional study, the level of susceptibility of the nurses to the ethical values was measured by the "Inclination to Ethical Values". The scale consists of 16 items and three dimensions (Love-Respect, Justice-Honesty, and Cooperation). The sample of the study was comprised of 122 nurses from the generation X and 115 nursing students from generation Y in public hospitals in Istanbul.

Results: While 81.1 % of the participants in the X-generation were female, 46.1 % of the participants in the Y generation were male, and the male gender was statistically significant (p = .003, p <.005). Education was low in both groups. All dimensions and total score of susceptibility to ethical values are higher in the X generation participants; the difference between total ethical values, propensity score, love–respect dimension, and cooperation dimension were statistically significant (p<0.05).

Conclusion: According to the results of the study, nurses in generation X are more inclination to the ethical values including love–respect and cooperation than nurses in generation Y. On the other hand, justice and honesty are common values of both generations. In the trainings to be given, it can be stated that it would be beneficial to focus on love–respect and cooperation issues.

Keywords: Ethics, ethical values, X and Y generation, nursing

Introduction

The word ethics is derived from the Greek word "ethos-ethikos." This word in Greek language system, principle, human behavior, tradition comes to the meaning (1). Our language is translated from the French word Éthique. Ethics is defined as the behaviors to be complied with or avoided by the parties in various professions (2). The word ethics comes from the Latin word Y arab ır, the word enek hulk Y and it is used to mean custom, habit, and good behavior (3). Ethics, as a word, is defined as a group of moral principles or values that regulate the behavior of the person or profession (4,5). In other words, it is expressed as the norms, ideals, principles, standards, or moral requirements that guide the conduct of human behavior and provide guidance on what to do or what not to do in professional studies (5–7).

Nurses, who are in constant contact with the patient in the health sector and who are the main employees of care and treatment, face ethical problems that they often find difficult to solve because of their expanding roles and responsibilities (8–12). Literature examines the ethical problems frequently encountered by nurses; in the care and treatment of patients, it is stated that there are different approaches with other members and institutions, protection of patient rights, care of patient in terminal period, receiving informed consent, sharing of limited resources, and non-ethical attitudes of colleagues (6,13–15). Nurses are expected to make the right decisions in the face of these ethical problems. However, in order for nurses to recognize ethical problems and make the right decisions at the stage of analysis, their tendency to ethical values defined as the ability to distinguish the ethical problem should be improved (16). Ethical decision-making, which is a complex process, requires to be ethical and sensitive to ethical values as well as ethical knowledge (12) In other words, ethical sensitivity is to solve ethical problems in all units that provide healthcare services, to clarify the problems, to justify the action, or to prevent an ethical dilemma (17). In this respect, as a professional member, nurses are expected to act according to ethical principles, laws, professional codes of ethics, and professional values while fulfilling their roles and responsibilities (10,15). In order to solve the ethical issues, the necessity of complying with some ethical principles, as well as the generational differences between the nurses involved in fulfilling these principles can be a significant problem. For this reason, it is necessary to know the reason of the differences in attitudes, behaviors, and behavior about ethical values and the characteristics of these generations. The average time frame for each generation is considered to be 15–20 years in the determination of generation distinctions. Today, the nursing workforce consists of three generations: the Baby Boom Generation (1946–1964), the generation X (1965–1980) and the generation Y, or the generation of the millennium (1981–2000) (18). Şen Bezirci and Kocaman (2013) showed that in a study conducted with 973 nurses in İzmir province, 5.3 % of the sample was in Infant Explosion, 50.5 % of them were X, and 44.2 % of them were in Generation Y (19). In this study, the characteristics of these two generations are as follows: Generation X has seen the birth of the computer and easily accepts the change (20). Working is part of their lives. Like the baby boom belt of the previous generation, "they do not live to work", "they work to live"; they attach importance to the family and work-life balance. They do not want to stay in jobs that do not meet their own requirements or are unable to progress (21). These generations of nurses are individualist in their business life. They know how to manage their time and their limits and complete their work without supervision; they are more result-oriented than the process (22). They are often hasty, want to be involved in decision-making processes, and care for their own program (23). Generation Y is a generation that is aware of its many options and its main characteristics are self-confidence (23). This generation is defined as a generation that acts without taking into account the results and wants many things right now. The most important feature in the development of Generation Y is the electronic environment. Instead of speaking face to face, e-mail or message writing is the preferred communication tool (24). Generation Y does not want to be a supervisor but mentor (21). Generation Y has been raised in a more child friendly environment than in previous generations. They are used to working and supervising teams according to the X generation. Managers working with them need to know that generation Y should have longer adaptation programs than the more independent generation X. If they cannot find what they expect in working environments, they are not afraid to change jobs (21).

Generation Y nurses consider themselves to have worked in this department for a long period of time after working in a department for two years. In addition, after five years and more working if they do not get promoted to leave; they think of going to an institution where they can rise rapidly e (23).

Considering the existing problems within the framework of ethics and health rights and the limitations of the studies in this field, it is a necessity to evaluate the perspectives of nurses, one of the cornerstones of health services, especially for x and y generation according to generation difference. Nowadays, there is a great need for nurses who can provide ethically sensitive and morally acceptable care. When faced with an ethically problematic situation, it is thought that understanding the behavior patterns of the x and y generation nurses will contribute to raising public health. For this reason, it was aimed to examine the difference between the levels of susceptibility of nurses in different generations to ethical values. Considering the inadequacy of the studies conducted on the subject, this study will make an important contribution to the susceptibility of nurses to ethical values.

Materials and Methods

Purpose and Type of Research

The study was designed as a descriptive and cross-sectional study. This study was conducted to determine the attitudes of the nurses in different generations to the ethical values and to determine their attitudes toward ethical values. To be in line with this aim, does x and y create a significant difference on the attitudes of nurses towards ethical values? created the question of research.

Research Universe and Sample

The research was conducted in two public hospitals operating in the European side of Istanbul during the period of January–March 2017. The sample of the study was carried out with 115 nursing students from generation Y and 122 nurses from X generation in the same hospitals. The universe of the study consisted of the nursing student and the working nurses at the time of the study in these two hospitals. Simple random sampling method was used in the study.

Data Collection Tools and Method

In order to measure students' attitudes toward ethical values, inclination to Ethics Values Scale was used, and demographic questions were asked to obtain personal information.

Personal information form: questions about demographic variables such as gender, age, education level, and ethics training of the participants' personal information.

The scale of Inclination to Ethics Values: The "Ethical Values Vulnerability Scale", which consists of 16 items that were validated by Kaya (2015), was prepared in 5-point Likert type. Scale items "1" totally disagree, "2" disagree, "3" I am undecided, "4" agree, and "5" is formed as totally agree. The scale consisted of three sub-factors: Factor – 1 Love, respect (1–8), Factor – 2 Justice, honesty (9–13), and Factor – 3 Cooperation (14–16). The Cronbach's Alpha value of the scale was 0.90 (25).

Data collecting: the data were distributed to the nurses by the researchers, the time for them to fill (2 days) was recognized and at the end of this period were collected by the researchers again.

Ethical Aspects of Research

In order to carry out the study, ethics committee permission and application number of 35218 dated January 2017 were obtained from the ethics committee of the university where the researchers were assigned. Before the data were collected, the participants were informed about the purpose of the study, the results would be used only for scientific purposes, the participation to the study was based on volunteering, the questions should be answered individually, and their verbal informed consent was obtained.

Analysis of Data

SPPS 23.0 statistical package program was used to evaluate the data. The distribution of the questions in the Personal Information Form was interpreted as frequency, percentage, and scale scores as mean, standard deviation. The normal distribution of the pre-analysis data with the Kolmogorov-Smirnov test was found to be normal. In the comparison of quantitative data, in the case of two groups, independent samples (independent samples) asında t in test were used for comparison of parameters between groups. Results were evaluated at 95 % confidence interval and p <0.05 significance level.

Result

While 81.1 % of the participants in the X generation were female sexes, 46.1 % of the participants in the Y generation were male and the difference was statistically significant (p: 003, p <.0.05). In addition, there was a statistically significant difference in the educational status and the mean age in both groups (p <.05). However, there was no significant difference for both groups in terms of obtaining professional ethics or ethical training (p> .0.05). Professional ethics or ethical education was found to be low in both groups.
(Tab. 1).

Tab. 1: Demographic Characteristics of Participants

Items	X generation nurse n(%)	Y generation nurse n(%)	P value
Male	23 (18.9)	53 (46.1)	*.003**
Female	99 (81.1)	62 (53.9)	
Married	86 (70.5)	6 (5.2)	*.043**
Single	36 (29.5)	109 (94.7)	
High school	14 (11.5)	115 (100)	*.004*
Associate Degree	22 (18.0)		
License	57(46.8)		
Master's Degree	29 (23.8)		
Obtaining professional ethics or ethics training	67 (54.9)	49 (42.6)	*.564**
Item	**X generation nurse (M ± SD)**	**Y generation nurse (M± SD)**	**P value**
Age	48.75 ± 9.55	23.75 ± 4.55	*.037*

M: Mean± SD. Standard Deviation.*Student's t-test, (*p<.001, **p<.005).X generation n=122, Y generation n=115.

Tab. 2: Comparison of Participants Score of Inclination to Ethics Values Scale

Items	X generation nurse (M ± SD)	Y generation nurse (M± SD	P value	t value
Love-respect	3,78± 0,72	2,68± 0,83	.013**	2.563
Justice-honesty	3,96± 0,80	3,06± 0,82	.028**	2,987
Cooperation	3,98± 0,93	2,98± 0,75	.034**	3.241
Total Score for Inclination to Ethical Values Scale	3,92± 0,72	2,32± 0,83	.004*	2,302

(*p<.001, **p<.005). Student's t-test,, M:Mean; SD: Standard Deviation

In order to determine whether the mean scores of the total score and sub-dimensions of the Inclination to Ethics Values Scale of the Nurses participating in the study showed a significant difference compared to the X generation and the Y generation nurses, the difference between the group means was statistically significant (p> 0.05). The difference was determined by the total score of all the subscales and the scale of the X generation. The total score and sub-dimension scores of the nurses working with generation X were found to be higher than those of nurses with Y generation.

Discussion and Conclusion

Ethical problems; they are in a complex structure that is not confined to a conscientious objection and prefer to choose the right or the wrong.. Therefore, it requires guidance and support and training in nurses working on appropriate approaches to the solution of ethical problems as well as in nurses who will take part in future working life (17). In the light of the data obtained in the study, while 81.1 % of nurses in the X-generation were female, 46.1 % of the participants in the Y generation were male, and the male gender was in the majority (p: 003, p <.0.05). This situation can be considered that the profession of nursing is no longer the profession of women, and that men in this profession will form the majority in the future.

In the study of Filizöz et al. (2015), it was observed that the nurses were predominantly between the young age group (46 % between the ages of 25–34) and the majority of study periods were between 1 and 5 years (35.7%) (10). Basak et al. (2010) reported that 67.8 % of nurses had occupational experience between 20 and 29 age group and 37.8 % between 1 and 5 years in their study to examine the ethical sensitivity of intensive care nurses (26). In our country, it is stated that the average age of the other nurses is low (27–30). In addition, the mean age of education was found to be significant in both groups, and there was a statistically significant difference (p <0.05). According to Akyol (2011) and Ertug et al. (2014), it was found out that nurses with undergraduate/graduate education had higher ethical sensitivities than those of Dikmen (2013) and Başak et al. (2010) found no significant relationship between education level and ethical sensitivity (9,15,16,26). These findings are partially similar to the results of our study, and this result may be thought to be due to the fact that the intern nurses have not completed their education yet and their average age is low.

Professional ethics and ethical education in the study no significant difference for both groups. (p > .0.05). Başak et al. (2010) reported that 51.7 % of nurses received postgraduate education in their studies in order to determine the ethical sensitivities of intensive care nurses (26). In the study which examined the ethical sensitivities of nurses working in İzmir province, they stated that they did not receive ethics training after graduation. In her study, Filizöz et al. (2015) found that ethics education was 69 % in the school age group and 31 % in the professional life group (10). These findings are similar to the results of our study and may suggest that ethics education is not considered in pre-graduate education and post-graduate in-service training.

Akyol (2011), Ertug et al. (2014) found out that nurses with undergraduate/graduate education had higher ethical sensitivities than those of Dikmen (2013) and Başak et al. (2010) found no significant relationship between education level and ethical sensitivity (9,15,16,26). Although ethics courses in undergraduate and postgraduate education and the awareness studies in this area are higher, it is thought that the ethical sensitivity of the undergraduate/graduate group is low in our study and this situation should be investigated more. In this study, it was found that the ethical sensitivities of the X-generation nurses and the Y-generation nurses were at a moderate level (3.92 ± 0.72, 2.32 ± 0.83).

As a result, it is recommended that there are no ethical dilemmas that may arise due to intergenerational differences, and ethical problems should be recognized and solved. In the trainings to be given, it can be stated that it would be beneficial to focus on love–respect and cooperation issues. In addition, it is considered that it is important to conduct studies in larger groups in order to determine the different variables that affect the ethic sensitivity of nurses.

Limitations of the Research

The study can only be considered as a limitation in the generalizability of the two public hospitals in Istanbul on the European side, as it is carried out with nurses.

Conflict of Interest

There is no conflict of interest by the authors.

Financial Disclosure

The authors declared that they did not receive financial support for this study.

References

1. Aktaş, K. (2014). Etik-Ahlak İlişkisi ve Etiğin Gelişim Süreci, *Uluslararası Yönetim ve Sosyal Araştırmalar Dergisi*, 1(2): 22–32.

2. Turkish Language Institution Dictionary (2019) http://www.tdk.gov.tr/index. php?option=com_bts&view=bts&kategori1=veritbn&kelimesec=1 18065,

3. Yaman, E., Çetinkaya Mermer, E. & Mutlugil, Ş. (2009). İlköğretim Okulu Öğrencilerinin Etik Davranışlara İlişkin Görüşleri: *Nitel Bir Araştırma, Değerler Eğitimi Dergisi*, 7 (17): 93–108.

4. Svensson G., & Wood, G. (2005). Corporate Ethics İn TQM: Management Versus Employee Expectations and Perceptions. *TQM Magazine*, 17(2):137–149.

5. Kutlay, O., & Yılmazlar, A. (2001). *Anestezi ve Yoğun Bakımda Etik*, Erdemir Demirhan (Ed.). Klinik Etik. Nobel Tıp Kitabevi: İstanbul.

6. Elçigil, A., Bahar, Z., Beşer, A., Mızrak, B., Bahçelioğlu, D., Demirtaş, D., Özdemir, D., Özgür, E., & Yavuz, H. (2011). Hemşirelerin Karşılaştıkları Etik İkilemlerin İncelenmesi. *Anadolu Hemşirelik ve Sağlık Bilimleri Dergisi*, 14(2): 52–60.

7. Kahriman, İ., & Çalık, K. Y.(2017). Klinik Hemşirelerin Etik Duyarlılığı. *Gümüşhane Üniversitesi Sağlık Bilimleri Dergisi*, 6(3): 111–121.

8. Aslan. Ö., Vural, H., & Avcı, P.Y. (2003). Ameliyathane Hemşirelerinin Etik Sorunlara Yönelik Yaklaşımlarının Belirlenmesi. *Gülhane Tıp Dergisi*, 45(2): 147–152.

9. Ertuğ, N., Aktaş, D., Faydali, S & Yalçın, O. (2014). Ethical Sensitivity and Related Factors of Nurses Working in the Hospital Settings. *Acta Bioethica*, 20 (2): 265–270.

10 .Filizöz, B., Mescib, G., Aşcıc, A., & Bağcıvan, E. (2015). Hemşirelerde Etik Duyarlılık: Sivas İli Merkez Kamu Hastanelerinde Bir Araştırma. *Türkiye İktisadi Girişim ve İş Ahlâkı Derneği İş Ahlakı Dergisi*, 8(1): 47–66.

11 .Dalcalı, B.K, Şendir, M. (2016). Hemşirelerin Kişisel Değerleri ile Etik Duyarlılıkları Arasındaki İlişkinin Belirlenmesi. *Florence Nightingale Hemşirelik Dergisi*, 24 (1): 1–9.

12. Utlu, N. (2016). Hastane Ortamında Hemşirelerin Etik Yaklaşımı ve Etik İkilemler. *İstanbul Aydın Üniversitesi Dergisi*, 29: 17–35.

13. Tang, P.F., Johansson, C., & Wadensten, B. (2007). Chinese Nurses' Ethıcal Concerns in a Neurologıcal Ward. *Nursing Ethics*, 14 (6): 810–824.

14. Austin, W., Kelecevic, J.,Goble, E. & Mekechuk, J. (2009). An Overview of Moral Distress and the Paediatric İntensive Care Team. *Nursing Ethics*, 16: 57–68.

15. Dikmen, Y. (2013). Yoğun Bakım Hemşirelerinde Etik Duyarlılığın İncelenmesi. *Cumhuriyet Hemşirelik Dergisi*, 2(1): 1–7.

16. Aksu, T. & Akyol, A. (2011). İzmir'deki Hemşirelerin Etik Duyarlılıklarının İncelenmesi. *Türkiye Klinikleri*, 19(1): 16–24.

17. Öztürk, H., Hintistan, S., Kasım, S., & Candaş, B. (2009). Yoğun Bakım Ünitelerinde Hekim ve Hemşirelerin Etik Duyarlılığı. *Yoğun Bakım Hemşireliği Dergisi*, 13(2): 77–84.

18. Sherman, R.O. (2006). Leading a Multigenerational Nursing Workforce: Issues, Challenges, and Strategies. OJIN: *The Online Journal of Issues in Nursing*, 11(2): p. 3

19. Şen Bezirci, S., & Kocaman, G. (2013). *Farklı Kuşaklardaki Hemşirelerin Meslekten ve İşten Ayrılma Niyetleri İle İş Doyumlarının İncelenmesi.* 1. Ulusal Hemşirelikte Yönetim Sempozyumu Kitabı, s;61. İstanbul.

20. Hart, S.M. (2006). Generational Diversity: Impact on Recruitment and Retention of Registered Nurses. *The Journal of Nursing Administration* 36(1): 10–12.

21. Carver, L., & Candela, L. (2008). Attaining Organizational Commitment across Different Generations of Nurses. *Journal of Nursing Management*, 16: 984–991.

22. Hendricks, J.M., & Cope, V.C. (2013). Generational Diversity: What Nurse Managers Need to Know. *Journal of Advanced Nursing*, 69(3): 717–725.

23. Clipper, B. (2012). Nurse Manager's Guide to an Intergenerational Workforce. SIGMA Theta Tau International, http:// site.ebrary.com/ id/10629217 (Date of access 30.01.2017).

24. Elçi M & Alpkan, L. (2009). The Impact of Perceived Organizational Ethical Climate on Work Satisfaction. *Journal of Business Ethics*, 84(3): 297–311.

25. Kaya, İ. (2015). Etik Değerlere Yatkınlık Ölçeği: Geçerlik Ve Güvenirlik Çalışması. *Journal of International Social Research*, 8(41): 968–974.

26. Başak, T., Uzun, Ş. & Arslan, F. (2010). Yoğun bakım hemşirelerinin etik duyarlılıklarının incelenmesi. *Gülhane Tıp Dergisi*, 52: 76–81.

27. Aytaç, N., Naharcı, H. ve Öztunç, G. (2008). Adana'da eğitim araştırma hastanelerinin yoğun bakım hemşirelerinde hastane enfeksiyonları bilgi düzeyi. Adnan *Menderes Üniversitesi Tıp Fakültesi Dergisi*, 9(3): 9–15.

28. Çelen, Ö. Karaalp, T., Kaya, S., Demir, C., Teke, A. & Akdeniz, A. (2007). Gülhane Askeri Tıp Fakültesi Eğitim Hastanesi yoğun bakım ünitelerinde görev yapan hemşirelerin uygulanan hizmet içi eğitim programlarından beklentileri ve bu programlar ile ilgili düşünceleri. *Gülhane Tıp Dergisi*, 49(1): 25–31.

29. Göz, F. & Gürelli Şalk, Ş. (2007). Yoğun bakım hemşirelerinin organ bağışı ile ilgili düşünceleri. *Fırat Sağlık Hizmetleri Dergisi*, 5(2): 77–88.

30. Aminu, I. M., & Shariff, M. N. M. (2014). Strategic Orientation, Access to Finance, Business Environment and SMEs Performance in Nigeria: Data Screening and Preliminary Analysis, *European Journal of Business and Management*, 6(35): 124–131.

Fadime Çınar and Fatma Eti Aslan

The Measurement of the Operating Room Nurses' Compassion Level: Turkish Validity and Reliability Study

Abstract: Objective: In this study, it was aimed to examine whether the Compassion Scale, which can measure the compassion for others with six dimensions, is a valid and reliable tool for the operating room nurses.

Material and Method: This methodological study was carried out with 236 nurses working in public and private hospitals between April and May 2017 in the European Side of Istanbul. In collecting the data, "Introductory Information Form" and "Compassion Scale", consisting of 6 dimensions of 24 items, were used to measure the compassion for others. For the scale, the validity of the subject was obtained by taking the opinions of the colleagues and by the expert evaluation. Item-total score correlation and Cronbach's alpha values were calculated for internal consistency/reliability. Exploratory and confirmatory factor analysis was performed for construct validity.

Results: The Cronbach Alpha value of the scale was found to be 0,821. Spearman-Brown coefficient was 0.813. As a result of the Basic Component Analysis, the factor loadings of all items were above the accepted value of 0,40. According to the Lawshe method, the scope validity values of all items were between 0.64–1.00 values above 0.59, which is the lower limit for 11 experts. According to confirmatory factor analysis, fit indexes of the scale (CFI = .97; NNFI = .96; SRMR = .05 and RMSEA = .06) were found.

Conclusion: According to the results of the study, it was determined that the Compassion Scale could be used as a valid and reliable scale in measuring the level of compassion of the operating room nurses.

Keywords: Nursing, care, compassion, validity, reliability

Introduction

The concept of compassion is defined as the motivation to help and empathize the individual who needs help in general (1–3). According to the Turkish Language Association, "is a feeling of sadness and pity because of the bad situation faced by one person or another creature" (4). Compassion with the combination of motivation, emotion, thought, and behavior; it is a cognitive process related to understanding the source of pain (5). In the literature, compassion is indicated as compassionate (sensitive) love, and it is stated as a behavioral, cognitive, and emotional attitude to support other people in times of need. Compassion– this includes behavior, empathy, and sympathy. Neff and Pommier (2013) stated that empathy and compassion are very similar and sometimes used interchangeably (6). However, in general, compassion and empathy are defined as different concepts (7). In addition, compassion is a more active reaction process to the troubled person. Besides, compassion as a common norm in almost every culture is an indicator of an individual virtue (8).

Nurses spend a long time with individuals who need help. Nurses have important roles in creating positive environments in care areas and accelerating recovery. They use compassion as a key to fulfill these roles (9). Moreover, the fact that nurses witness the most vulnerable and special situations of the individuals they care for causes the compassionate care to come to the fore (8,10–13). Compassionate care is a holistic approach model that increases patient satisfaction, has positive physiological effects on the patient, and accelerates the recovery (14).

In the provision of health services, mutual trust, respect, effective communication, and cooperation with the patients and their families provide compassionate care. The compassionate presentation of patient care is expected from all health workers. In the literature, compassionate care practices; It has also been emphasized that it affects the management of symptoms positively in operating rooms, surgical clinics, intensive care units, and all other long-term care settings (14). However, bringing compassion and empathy can also cause negative effects on those who feel compassion (8).

Empathy for a patient may cause the individual to think of himself as a patient. This negative effect can lead to occupational burnout, especially in the areas of professionalism that continue to work between the concepts of compassion and empathy, such as nursing (11,12,15). The concept of compassion must be managed in order to prevent the level of occupational burnout from being unwanted due to empathy and therefore compassion. In order to manage the concept of compassion, factors affecting the level of compassion should be measured. In order to find and manage the factors affecting compassion, there is a need to measure the levels of compassion. In order to measure the level of compassion in the operating room nurses, who are involved in surgical interventions where trauma, pain, and suffering process is low or not, patient studies are not yet sufficient (14). Therefore, in this study, it was examined whether The Compassion Scale, which can measure the compassion for others with six dimensions, is a valid and reliable tool for operating room nurses. This study is thought to fill this gap in the literature.

Materials and Methods

Objective

In this study, it was aimed to examine whether the Compassion Scale, which can measure the compassion for others with six dimensions, is a valid and reliable tool for the operating room nurses

The Universe and Sample of Research

This methodological study was carried out between April-May 2017. The universe of the study completed at least one year in the public and private hospitals operating in the European side of Istanbul in the beginning of 2017 and operated nurses (N = 493). No sampling method was used in the study and all of the universe was included in the study (16). However, 214 nurses did not want to participate in the study. Forty-three participants who did not fully answer the questions in the Compassion Scale were excluded. For this reason, 236 nurses were included in the sample.

Data Collection Tools and Data Collection

Research data: Obtained by face-to-face survey method with "Introductory Information Form" and "Compassion Scale" to collect demographic information of operating room nurses participating in the study.

"Introductory Information Form : It consists of questions suchas age, education, gender, professional experience, marital status.

Compassion Scale: Developed by Pommier (17), adapted to Turkish by the Akdeniz and the Deniz (1), and , and able to measure compassion for others by six dimensions Kindness (6,8,16,24), Indifference (2,12,14,18), Common Humanity (11,15,17,20), Separation (3,5,10,22), Mindfulness (4,9,13,21), and Disengagement (1,7,19,23) 24-item – It is a 5-point Likert-type scale. Scoring of items in scale, 1 = Never, 2 = Rarely, 3 = Occasional 4 = Frequent, 5 = Always. It is calculated by inverting the scores of the sub-dimensions of indifference, separation nd disengagement. The lowest possible score is 24, and the highest score is 120. As the score from the scale increases, the level of compassion of the operating room nurses is increasing.

As a result of the confirmatory factor analysis (CFA) performed by the Akdeniz and Deniz (1) the existence of six dimensions constituting the structure of the scale was confirmed. The Cronbach Alpha internal consistency reliability coefficient for the whole scale was .85. Factor loads of the sub-dimensions of the scale;

for the sub-dimension of kindness .61–.74, .56–.69 for indifference, .54–.83 for common humanity, .51–.73 separation, .55–.72 for mindfulness, and .58–.68 for disengagement from ıt ranges. The fit indices of the scale (CFI = .97; NNFI = .96; SRMR = .05 and RMSEA = .06) were found. The internal consistency reliability coefficients ranged from .57 to .77 for sub-dimensions. In the validity and reliability study of the Turkish version, it was determined that the English form scores of 41 people who have mastered English and Turkish languages and the Turkish form scores re-applied after 25 days were r = .78 (p <.01).

The reliability of the scale was assessed by item analysis, internal consistency, and time-invariance (test-retest). The repetition of the test was repeated by 30 participants twice in 2 weeks. These results were consistent with the findings obtained from the Akdeniz and the Deniz (1) and the scale was determined as six dimensions and 24 items. For the purpose of this study, the language validity of the scale was not done again because of the validity and reliability of the Turkish version. However, the suitability of the scope was evaluated by the experts in the scope of the Turkish culture and it was questioned whether there were any questions that could not be understood by the pilot study. The Turkish version of the scale was consistent.

Scope Validity of the Scale

The scope validity of the scale was determined according to the Lawshe method. For the content validity, 4 faculty members from the Department of Internal Medicine Nursing were informed to 4 faculty members from the Department of Human and Society, 2 operating room nurses, and 1 measurement and evaluation specialist. A form was prepared for expert opinions. In this form, which is sent to the experts by e-mail, (a) each item measures the targeted structure (b) the substance is related to the structure but is unnecessary, (c) the substance is graded as not measuring the targeted structure. In this method, the scope validity rates of the experts were gathered by collecting their opinions about any item. Coverage validity ratios were obtained by the lack of a ratio of the number of experts stating say necessary toplam opinion of any item to the total number of experts indicating the opinion of the article[18]. According to the expert opinion, the Turkish version was not understood and the items needed were to be corrected. During the pilot application, the participants had difficulty in understanding the questions.

Data Analysis

Test-retest, Cronbach Alpha internal consistency, and Spearman-Brown (Split Half) coefficients were examined for the reliability of the scale, and confirmatory factor analysis was performed. For the reliability of the scale, the Lawshe (18,19) method and the Basic Component Analysis were performed. Scope Validity Ratio was examined and evaluated by 6 field experts and 5 academicians. In the Basic Component Analysis, factor load, KMO (Kaiser-Meyer-Olki and Barletsüs Test of Sphericity tests were performed. All analyzes were performed in SPSS 17.0 for Windows (SPSS Inc., Chicago, IL, USA) with a 95 % confidence interval. The distribution of the questions in the Personal Information Form was interpreted as frequency, percentage, and scale scores as mean, standard deviation. Results were evaluated at 95 % confidence interval and p <0.05 significance level.

Ethical Aspects of Research

Ethics committee approval was obtained from the research institution. In order to implement the study, hospital administrations were contacted and information about the study was given and written permission was obtained. Participants received written and verbal consent to participate in the study.

Results

Demographic Characteristics of the Participants

In the study the nurses participating were 27.1 % of male and 72.9 % of female. The nurses were 60.2 % of 30 years and under 22.5 % 31–40 years old between, 10.2 % between 41–50 years old, 7.2 % were 5 years and over. 42.8 % of nurses had experience between 1–5 years, 18.6 % between 6–10 years, 19.1 % between 10–15 years, and 19.5 % had 15 years and more experience. 69.5 % of all nurses were married and 30.5 % were single. The mean scores of the tablo Compassion Scale of the operating room nurses are given in Tab. 1.

Tab. 1: The Mean Score of the Operating Room Nurses Compassion Scale (N 236)

	Mean	S.D	Min.	Max.
Kindness	3,68	0,72	4	20
Indifference	3,96	0,80	4	20
Common Humanity	3,98	0,93	4	20
Separation	3,32	0,72	4	20
Mindfulness	3,52	0,83	4	20
Disengagement	3,38	0,75	4	20
Compassşon Scale Total	3,92	0,82	24	120

M: Mean, ± S.D. Standard Deviation

In Tab. 1, the mean size of "Kindness Subscale" was (3,68 ± 0,72), and the mean of the "Indifference Subscale" (3,96 ± 0,80). ± 0,93), " Common Humanity Subscale" average (3,98 ± 0,93); Separation Subscale" average (3,32 ± 0,72), Mindfulness Subscale average (3,52 ± 0,83); Disengagement Subscale" average (3,38 ± 0,75). The mean of Compassion Scale Total (3.92 ± 0.82) was found.

Lawshe Method Validity

According to the Lawshe method, the scope validity rates of all items were higher than the lower limit of 0.59 for 11 experts and between 0.64 and 1.00. The scope validity value of the article. Only suffering is a common experience for all people that the KGO value of the substance is 0.64 and above the limit value. Item Analysis and Factor Structure of the Scale

The item analysis of the scale was performed before construct validity analysis. Total score correlations of 24 items in the scale were examined. The item-total correlation coefficients of the scale were found to be r = 0.37 to 0.68, positive and statistically significant. Principal Component Analysis was performed for the determination of factor structure. Kaiser-Meyer Olkin (KMO) coefficient of the scale was 0.76 and the result of Barlett test was $X^2 = 3223,652$; p = 0.000 (p <0.05). The first factor analysis was carried out and the scale was composed of 7 sub-dimensions. However, in this first analysis, it was decided to keep the score at the highest point since the difference between the factors in which some items were in more than one dimension and the difference between them was greater than 0.10. After this process, it was determined that 24-item scale was collected in 6 sub-dimensions by using varimax perpendicular rotation technique. The total variance of the 6 factors determined was 51.480 %. The amount of variance explained by the factors; It was determined that 22.795 % of the kindness factor, 13.526 % of the ındifference factor, 7.338 % of the common humanity factor, 7.623 % of the separation factor, 5.098 mindfulness, % 7.623 of the disengagement factor. Factor loads of these six dimensions were found to range; for kindness dimension, .45–.65 for indifference, .58–79 for indifference, .45–.64 Common Humanity, .64–.72 for Separation, .58.76 for Mindfulness, and. .71–.85 for Disengagement.The fit indices of the scale (CFI = .98; NNFI = .97; SRMR = .05 and RMSEA = .07) were determined. The internal consistency reliability coefficients were found to vary between .64 and .77 for sub-dimensions. The internal consistency coefficient of the scale was Cronbach's alpha value of 0.821. Factor loads and factor loadings are shown in Tab. 3 as a result of factor analysis.

Tab. 2: Results of the Lawshe Analysis Conducted for Scope Validity (1)

	Required	Not Required	Scope Validation Rate Value
1. When people cry in front of me, I often don't feel anything at all..	11		1,00
2. Sometimes when people talk about their problems, I feel like I don't care.	10	1	0,82
3. I don't feel emotionally connected to people in pain.	10	1	0,82
4. I tend to listen patiently when people tell me their problems.	10	1	0,82
5. I can't really connect with other people when they're suffering.	11		1,00
6. If I see someone going through a difficult time, I try to be caring toward that person.	11		1,00
7. I don't think much about the concerns of others.	11		1,00
8. When others feel sadness, I try to comfort them..	10	1	0,82
9. I pay careful attention when other people talk to me	10	1	0,82
10. When I see someone feeling down, I feel like I can't relate to them.	10	1	0,82
11. Everyone feels down sometimes, it is part of being human.	11		1,00
12. When others are feeling troubled, I usually let someone else attend to them..	11		1,00
13. I notice when people are upset, even if they don't say anything.	11		1,00
14. Sometimes I am cold to others when they are down and out.	10	1	0,82
15. It's important to recognize that all people have weaknesses and no one's perfect..	10	1	0,82
16. I like to be there for others in times of difficulty..	10	1	0,82
17. Despite my differences with others, I know that everyone feels pain just like me.	10	1	0,82
18. I don't concern myself with other people's problems..	11		1,00
19. I often tune out when people tell me about their troubles.	11		1,00

(continued on next page)

Tab. 2: (continued)

	Required	Not Required	Scope Validation Rate Value
20. I don't concern myself with other people's problems..	9	2	0,64
21. When people tell me about their problems, I try to keep a balanced perspective on the situation	11		1,00
22. I feel detached from others when they tell me their tales of woe.	11		1,00
23. I try to avoid people who are experiencing a lot of pain..	10	1	0,82
24. My heart goes out to people who are unhappy.	10	1	0,82

In order to test the internal consistency within the scope of reliability, Chronbach Alpha values were examined. The total Cronbach Alpha value of the scale was 0.821. The sub-dimensions of the scale include Cronbach's Alpha values, Kindness; 0.76, Indifference; 0.72, 3. Common Humanity; 0.75, Separation 0.71. Mindfulness; 0.79 and Disengagement; 0,81.The relationship between the scale and its sub-dimensions was evaluated by the Spearman-Brown correlation analysis technique and a statistically significant positive correlation was found between the total score and all sub-dimension scores of the scale ($p < 0.001$ and $p < 0.005$) (Tab. 4).

Time-invariance (test-retest): For repetition of the test, 30 subjects were administered twice with 2 weeks intervals. Pearson correlation value was 0.76 ($p = 0.0009$).

Discussion

In this study, it was evaluated whether The Compassion Scale adapted to Turkish by Akdeniz and Deniz (1) was valid in determining the level of compassion of the operating room nurses. Factor analysis and content (content) validity, item-total score correlation, internal consistency and time invariance methods were used in this evaluation. Also, the suitability of the Turkish culture was examined by the experts during the scope validity. Validity is a measure of whether a test or scale actually measures the feature it wants to measure. For this purpose, if a scale measures the feature it wants to measure correctly, it is considered valid. A valid scale must also be reliable. Reliability is defined as consistency between participants' responses to scale items (20).

Tab. 3: Factor Loads and Factor Groups of Scale İtems

	Kindness	Indifference	Common Humanity	Separation	Mindfulness	Disengagement
C_6	,551					
C_8	,656					
C_16	,588					
C_24	,457					
C_2		-,589				
C_12		,798				
C_14		,675				
C_18		,630				
C_11			,550			
C_15			,641			
C_17			,448			
C_20			,592			
C_3				,735		
C_5				,625		
C_10				,741		
C_22				-,644		
C_4					,766	
C_9					-,314	
C_13					,642	
C_21					-,580	
C_1						-,715
C_7						,725
C_19						,795
C_23						,853

KMO: 0,764 X^2: 3223,652 p<0,005

The Lawsh method was used for the scope validity of the scale. Again in the Lawshe method, the validity levels of all items are above the value of the .40 factor load accepted in the literature and the Scope validity value determined for 11 experts (18,19). Therefore, the scale was found to be sufficient to measure the level of compassion of the operating room nurses. It was determined that there was consensus among experts by taking expert opinion for the scope validity and that the scale expressions were appropriate for our culture and represent the perception of compassion for the operating room nurses.

Tab. 4: Correlation Analysis of Scale Dimensions

Faktörler	Mean	S.D	1	2	3	4	5	6
Kindness	3,68	0,72	1					
Indifference	3,96	0,80	,024	1				
Common Humanity	3,98	0,93	,054	,385**	1			
Separation	3,32	0,72	, 454**	,177**	,212**	1		
Mindfulness	3,52	0,83	,367**	,259**	,118*	,479**	1	
Disengagement	3,38	0,75	,467*	,383**	,279**	,128*		1
Cronbach Alpha Reliability Coefficient	0,76	0,72	0,75	0,71	0,79	81		

* <0.001, **p<0.005

In order to determine the factor structure, it was found that the items were collected under six factors reflecting the level of compassion of the operating room nurses and consisted of 24 items. These factors are kindness, indifference, common humanity, separation, mindfulness, and disengagement. According to Burnell and Agan (2013) in the first place on the scale where the patients evaluated the compassionate nurse behaviors, 1. Passing the pain, 2. Understanding the medical problems, 3. The nurse is professionally sufficient, 4. The ability to work within the team, 5. The practice of treating patients without judging is defined as compassionate behavior (21).

According to Neff's (2003) model, compassionate focuses on three dimensions. These dimensions are: 1. Goodness, 2. Common feelings of humanity, 3. It is defined as accepting people without judgment, as they are (22,23). Chambers and Ryder (2009) merciful care; with six basic components: 1. Empathy and sensitivity, 2. Dignity and respect, 3. Listening and response, 4. Cultural diversity and competence, 5. Elections and priorities, 6. Empowerment and defense (23). Van der Cingel (2011) in his study; it has a structure that is acceptable with at least seven dimensions of compassion (24). Compassion in nursing and patient communication is a tool that supports the professional process. These results show similar dimensions with the factor structure of the scale adapted to Turkish by Akdeniz and Deniz (1), and the level of compassion of the operating room nurses.

Although there are many methods used to test the reliability, the most commonly used are substance analysis, internal consistency, and time invariance (25). In the literature, it is stated that substances with a item-total correlation of 0.30 and higher distinguish the feature to be measured at the best degree. In this study, the item-total correlation values of the scale items were above 0.30, indicating that the discriminative power of the substances was good (26). It can be said that the scale items distinguish well from the mercy levels of the operating room nurses.

Another measure that assesses the reliability of a scale is internal consistency. The most commonly used Cronbach Alpha reliability coefficient for evaluating internal consistency. Cronbach Alpha coefficient less than 0.40 is not reliable, it is very reliable between 0,40–0,59, it is highly reliable between 0,60–0,79, and it is highly reliable between 0,80–1,00 (16,20). In this study, the Cronbach Alpha coefficient of the Compassion Scale was 0.82 for the operating room nurses and had a good degree of reliability. In the study of Akdeniz and Deniz (2016), the Cronbach's Alpha value of the scale was 0.85 and Çingöl et al. (2018) found Cronbach's Alpha value to be 0.87 (1,13). The reliability results of this study are consistent with the literature. The reliability results of this study are consistent with the literature.

Another feature of a measuring instrument to be reliable is that it provides consistent results in repeated measurements. The most commonly used method is the test-retest method. The results of the two applications are evaluated by correlation analysis. The closer the correlation coefficient is to 1, the better is the time invariance of the test (20, 27). In this study, the correlation coefficient obtained by the test-re-test method is 0.76. This result shows that there is a strong relation between the measurements of the Compassion Scale in two separate times and shows the invariance of the scale according to time.

Result

Patient satisfaction levels can be increased with compassionate care practices that may be a quality indicator. By increasing the comfort of care, the patient can feel himself well. Therefore, there is a need to develop awareness about the concept of compassion and compassionate care, which are not subject to sufficient studies in the field of nursing. According to the results of this study, it is a valid and reliable measurement instrument of compassion scale in measuring the level of compassion of the operating room nurses. It can be said that the average score of the operating room nurses from the scale is high.

In the area of nursing, studies can be repeated to address the dimensions of compassion more comprehensively in a more diverse and larger sample. The concept of compassionate care – in-service trainings to graduate nurses and student nurses can be adopted with compassionate care issues added to renewed curriculum programs. Thus, it is thought that the sense of compassion will be developed and put into practice. In addition, measurement of the concept of compassion, which may cause the occupational burnout of nurses in field applications, supporting the in-service trainings and making awareness raising studies in this field can help to achieve positive gains in field applications.

Limitations of the Research

The study is limited to the opinions of 236 operating room nurses working in private hospitals operating in the European side of Istanbul in 2017 and the data obtained from scale items.

Conflict of Interest

There is no conflict of interest by the authors.

Financial Disclosure

The authors declared that they did not receive financial support for this study.

References

1. Akdeniz, S., & Deniz, M.E. (2016). Merhamet ölçeği'nin Türkçeye uyarlanması: geçerlik ve güvenirlik çalışması. *The Journal of Happiness & Well-Being.* 4(1): 50–61.

2. Cingel, M. (2011). Compassion in Care: A Qualitative Study of Older People with a Chronic Disease and Nurses. *Nursing Ethics.* 18(5): 672–685.

3. Dietze, E.V., & Orb, A. (200). Compassionate Care: A Moral Dimension of Nursing. *Nursing Inquiry.* 7(3): 166–174.

4. Turkish Language Institution Dictionary http://www.tdk.gov.tr/, (Date of access: 16.01.2018)

5. Gilbert, P. (2005). Compassion and Cruelty: A Biopsychosocial Approach. In P. Gilbert (Ed), *Compassion: Conceptualisations, Research and Use in Psychotherapy.* (pp.9–74). London, England: Routledge.

6. Neff, K.D., & Pommier, E. (2013). The Relationship between Self-Compassion and Other-Focused Concern among College Undergraduates, Community Adults, and Practicing Meditators. *Self and Identity.* 12, 160–176.

7. Gladkova, A. (2010). Sympathy, Compassion, and Empathy in English and Russian: A Linguistic and Cultural Analysis. *Culture & Psychology.* 16, 267–285.

8. Hökelekli H. (2013). Merhamet. *Dem Dergi.* 1(4), 78–82.

9. Neff, K.D. (2004). Self-Compassion and Psychological Well-Being. *Constructivism in the Human Sciences.* 9(2): 27–37.

10. Atilla, G. (2015). Merhamet etmenin dayanılmaz ağırlığı: hemşirelerde merhamet yorgunluğu. *Süleyman Demirel Üniversitesi İktisadi ve İdari Bilimler Fakültesi Dergisi.*20: 299–313.

11. Dikmen, Y., & Aydın, Y., Tabakoğlu, P. (2016). Compassion Fatigue: A Study of Critical Care Nurses in Turkey. *Journal of Human Sciences.* 13(2): 2879–2884.

12. Şirin, M., & Yurttaş A. (2015). Hemşirelik bakımının bedeli: merhamet yorgunluğu. Dokuz Eylül Üniversitesi Hemşirelik Fakültesi Elektronik Dergisi 2015; 8(2): 123–130.

13. Çingöl, N., Çelebi, E., Zengin, S., & Karakaş, M. (2018). Bir Sağlık Yüksekokulu Hemşirelik Bölümü Öğrencilerinin Merhamet Düzeylerinin İncelenmesi. *Klinik Psikiyatri Dergisi,* 21(1):61-67

14. Uğurlu, A.K., & Eti Aslan, F. (2017). Merhamet ve Hemşirelik: Merhamet Ölçülebilir mi? *Turkiye Klinikleri Hemsirelik Bilimleri,* 9(3): 233–238.

15. İkiz, F.E. (2010). Psikolojik danışmanların tükenmişlik düzeylerinin incelenmesi. *Ahi Evran Üniversitesi Egitim Fakültesi Dergisi* .11(2): 25–43.

16. Sümbüloğlu, K. ve Sümbüloğlu, V. Biyoistatistik.11.Baskı. Ankara.Hatipoğlu Basım ve Yayım.2005.

17. Pommier E.A. (2011). The Compassion Scale. Dissertation Abstracts International Section A: *Humanities and Social Sciences.* 72: 1174.

18. Lawshe C.H. (1975). A Quantitative Approach to Content Validity. *Personnel Psychology.* 28: 563–575.

19. Yurdugül, H. (2005). *Ölçek Geliştirme çalışmalarında kapsam geçerliliği için kapsam geçerlilik indekslerinin kullanılması.* XIV. Ulusal Eğitim Bilimleri Kongresi Kitabı. 1–5, Denizli.

20. Çakmur, H. (2012). Araştırmalarda Ölçme- Güvenilirlik-Geçerlilik. TAF Preventive *Medicine Bulletin.* 11(3): 339–344

21. Burnell, L., Agan, D.L. (2013). Compassionate Care: Can It Be Defined and Measured? The Development of the Compassionate Care Assessment Tool. *International Journal of Caring Sciences.* 6(2):180–187.

22. Neff, K.D. (2003). The Development of Validation of a scale to measure self compassion. Self and Identity. 2(3): 223–250.

23. Bhartendra, S., Triza, J. (2015). Self-Compassion: Basis of Quality Nursing Care. *Asian J. Nursing Edu. and Research.* 5(2): 279–282.

24. van der Cingel, M. (2011). Compassion in Care: A Qualitative Study of Older People with a Chronic Disease and Nurses. *Nurs Ethics.* 18(5): 672–685.

25. Saydam, B.K., Çeber, E., Bilge, A., Can, Ö.H., Mermer, G., Demirelöz, M., et al. (2010). Reliability and Validity of the Reproductive Health Scale for Turkish Adolescents. *Turkiye Klinikleri J Med Sci.* 30(2): 659–668.

26. Büyüköztürk Ş. (2016). *Sosyal bilimler için veri analizi el kitabı.* Ankara, Pegem Akademi

27. Şencan, H. (2005). *Geçerlilik ve Güvenilirlik.* 1. Baskı. Ankara: Seçkin Yayıncılık; p.355–414.

FatmaEti Aslan, SemraBulbuloglu, and IlknurYayla

The Intra-Operative Care Safety Study: Medical Errors in the Operating Room

Abstract: Background: Patient safety is an important part of intra-operative care because some patients may be more vulnerable. Medical errors may lead to various injuries. **Objective:** It is aimed to observe the medical errors inthe operating room and determine the practices of healthcare nurses in case of mistakes and their needs of information.

Methods: The descriptive study was carried out at a state hospital in Turkey inJune 2016 and involved 42 operating room nurses, as well as observing 339 operations. The validity of the healthcare practices was compared. The data were collected via the observation method and recorded on data forms. We counted the percentage scores for each dimension of patient safety culture and assessed the factors contributing to patient safety errors.

Results: 42 professionals, six types of surgery, 339 operations and six dimensions of patient safety were observed and divided into nine contributing factors. The most common medical errors were in abdominal surgery by 23.18 %, the most frequently stated dimensions were patient diagnosis, and intervention safety by 31.96 %, the most effective contributing factor that increased the probability of making mistakes was lack of experience, knowledge, and training by 32.42 %. **Conclusion:** In health care, adverse events constitute a high risk or reducing the quality of care. Precautions should be taken for patient safety principles to an optimal level by individuals, institutions, and states.

Keywords: Operating room, patient, patient safety, safety

Introduction

In recent years, the concept of patient safety has been commonly discussed extensively in the literature on medicine and nursing, and it is one of the most important requirements for healthcare[1-4]. Surgery is quite risky for peri-operative teams[1]. Therefore, the members of the surgical team should reduce these risks by taking preventive measures for patient safety.

Prevention of possible risks, deterioration of current situation, and development of new problems after hospitalization, as well as not delaying discharge, and preservation of patient information are involved in the contents of patient safety principles[1,2].

Patient safety in the operating room (OR) plays a key role in providing high-quality health care. To prevent injury and infections, successful communication, effective patient diagnosis and intervention, accurate management of surgical pathology specimens, and correct record-keeping are sub dimensions of ensuring patient safety in the operating room[1,5,6]. In the United States more than 400,000 deaths occur every year because of medical errors[7]. In literature reviews, it was observed that medical errors originate from faulty healthcare practices and are based on foundations of systems and organization[2,3,8]. Approximately 40 % of undesired events occur in the OR, and 50 % of such cases are preventable[7]. 44 % of these events lead to prolonged stay atthe hospital, and 8.7 % result in permanent damage or death[9].

This study aimed to observe the medical errors in the operating room and the contributing factors.

Methods

Design

The study protocol was approved by the Adiyaman Clinical Research Ethics Committee with the decision dated 25 May 2016 and numbered 2016/4–2. The study used a questionnaire and a socio-demographic information form, which assessed the participants' medical error statuses. We observed the medical errors, their causes and management, as well as the effectiveness of such causes in the operating room. The descriptive study was realized between June 1 and 30 2016 at a research and training hospital in Turkey and comprised operating room nurses. After the approval from the ethics committee and the hospital's management, a data-collection form was prepared by researchers, and it comprised two parts. The first part included questions on patient safety under 6 headings and descriptive information about the OR nurses. The second part evaluated the factors that contribute to medical errors, dimensions of patient safety, and factors that contribute to patient safety under 9 headings. In this study, 339 operations in abdominal surgery, head, neck and face surgery, orthopedic cases, thoracic surgery, genitourinary cases, and cardiovascular surgery were observed. The data were collected via the observation method and recorded on data forms.

Participants

A total of 42 nurses were included in this study. This observational study used a prospective review of the medical errors about patient safety in the operating room. Practices related to patient safety were obtained from the participating nurses at a research and training hospital in Turkey. The nurses who volunteered to participate were included.

Tab. 1: Demographic Characterization of Patient and Errors by Classification

Operation type	Age in Years					Gender of the Patients		Types of Errors on Operations (%)						
	<18	18to30	30 to 45	45 to 60	>60	Female	Male	P.I.	S.C.	P.D.I.S.	I.C.	S.P.S.S.	R.S.	Total
Abdominal surgery	7	13	5	7	12	18	26	2.88	6.4	6.3	1.3	1.9	4.4	23.18
Head, neck, face surgery	16	14	27	24	38	74	45	4.7	5.6	5.4	0.2	1.1	4.2	21.2
Orthopedia cases	23	16	13	9	26	53	34	2.98	3.3	5.4	0.3	0.6	3.4	15.98
Thoracic surgery	0	1	6	4	12	13	10	0.41	6.3	7.6	0.4	0.4	4.1	19.21
Genitourinary cases	26	11	3	2	10	16	36	1.18	1.4	3.1	0.3	0.2	4.2	10.38
Cardio-vascular surgery	-	-	-	4	10	3	11	2.1	0.85	4.16	0.15	0.1	2.67	10.03
Total	72	55	54	50	108	177	162	14.25	23.85	31.96	2.65	4.3	22.9	99.98

P.I.:To prevent injury, S.C.:Safe communication, P.D.I.S:Patient diagnosis and intervention safety, I.C.:Infection control,S.P.S.S.:Surgicalpathology specimen safety, R.S.:Registration safety

Tab. 2: Patient Safety in the OR by Taxonomy

Patient Safety Classification	Errors[a] (%) n=2603
To prevent injury	(14.25)371
Safe communication	(23.85) 621
Patient diagnosis and intervention safety	(31.96) 832
Infection control	(2.65) 69
Surgical pathology specimen safety	(4.3) 112
Registration safety	(22.97) 598
[a]It's possible that an error affected more than one contributing factor	

Data Collection

Operation selection was stratified with the aim of reaching a range of procedures. A comparison was made between the patient safety practices of the OR nurses and the guidelines of the Association of Peri-Operative Registered Nurses (AORN) on patient safety standards[1,6]. The technical and non-technical skills for patient safety interventions expected from nurses and the medical errors in the OR were recorded and compared.

Data Analysis

The data that were obtained in this study were evaluated using the SPSS for Windows 17 package software. Records, observational results, and questionnaire responses were collected, and the results were tabulated. The socio-demographic characteristics of the nurses were used for the calculations, and the results were analyzed in terms of frequencies and percentages.

Findings

In this observational study with 42 nurses, we found that the meanage of the nurses was 35.61 years (SD=3.66), 95.24 % of the participants were working staff nurses, 17.5 % were trained on patient safety in the OR, and 59.5 % had experience of five years or more. In this study, a total of 339 operations were observed (Tab. 1), with 2603 recorded medical errors, almost all of which were regarded preventable and non-fatal (Tab. 2,3). The most common medical errors were defined in abdominal surgery by 23.18 % and head, neck, and face surgery by 21.2 % (Tab. 1). Lack of experience, knowledge, oreducation was the most common issues that led to medical errors in the OR for the participations. Communication problems had a generally important influence on medical errors

Tab. 3: Types of Safety Issues by Dimension of Patient Safety in the OR

Patient Safety Dimension in the OR	Errors n= 2603	%
To Prevent Injury	**371**	**14.25**
• Safe transfer of the patient to an from operating room	20	0.76
• Ideal patient positioning to prevent injury also surgical and anaesthetic team members for easy access patient positioning by informed staff	50	1.92
• Need to position changing more than two hours operations	11	0.42
• An evaluation of skin condition has been made for pressure ulcer, injury, erythema, or redness, rubbish.	290	11.14
Safe communication	**621**	**23.85**
• The patient is greeted with name in the operating room by nurses.	185	7.1
• Operating room nurses identify themselves.	196	7.52
• Full communication for patients having optical, audition, speaking or language issues.	3	0.11
• Patient introduce has been checked in the pre-operative process.	34	1.3
• Patient respectability and comfort is proved as far as possible along the patients intraoperative process.	203	7.79
Patient diagnosis and intervention safety	**832**	**31.96**
• Complete patients record laboratory investigate and X-rays are present.	64	2.45
• Pre-operative special preparation has been checked for surgery (bowel preparation, catheter present etc.).	23	0.88
• To mark surgical region by distinctly.	62	2.38
• To interrogated allergy record.	42	1.61
• To checkpre-medication status	57	2.18
• To explore pace maker and other implants present.	72	2.76
• To use(if necessary) clippers or depilatory cream	5	0.19
• To check last time the patient catering.	41	1.57
• To measurement and record the patient VİTAL signs.	127	4.87
• Continually monitoring for body temperature with appropriate technique.	339	13,02
Infection control	**69**	**2.65**
• Surgical team has been liable to the patient about aseptic technique.	19	0.72
• Before the surgical incision, the patient skin preparation with aseptic technique and to prevent pooling, using an appropriate solution.	38	1.45

(continued on next page)

Tab. 3: (continued)

Patient Safety Dimension in the OR	Errors n= 2603	%
• If there is a wound the patient, wound dressing prior to operation.	12	0.46
Surgical Pathology Specimen Safety	**112**	**4.3**
• Surgical pathology specimen management safety	112	4.30
Registration safety	**598**	**22.97**
• Complete registration in detail	246	9.45
• Appropriate using of surgical safety checklist	237	9.1
• To control instructed consent and letter of acceptance	19	0.72
• In the absence of perioperative team member, all practice delivered will be reported, such as drains, care interventions, all records, catheters, the patient's, implants.	96	3.68

Tab. 4: Patient Safety Errors in the OR by Contributing Factors

Patient Safety Errors of Contributing Factors	
Contributing Factors	**Errors[a](%), n=2603**
Communication problems	803 (30.84)
Staff in caution	136 (5.22)
Lack of experience, knowledge, education	844 (32.42)
Lack of guideline, protocols, policies	36 (1.38)
Intense work pressure	47 (1.8)
Staff deficiency	42 (1.61)
Poor awareness to staff	124(4.76)
Environmental problems	226(8.68)
Other issues (documentation issues, in adequate ingredients, poor organization etc.)	345(13.25)

[a]It's possible that an error affected more than one contributing factor

(Tab. 4). The most frequent error dimensions were patient diagnosis and intervention safety by 31.96 % and communication safety by 23.85 %. Medical errors were defined in all dimensionsin the procedures during the intra-operative process, and significantly at the patient diagnosis and intervention, communication, and registration stages.

Discussion

This study revealed the most frequent medical errors in intra-operative care in a large number of operations on patients (2603 medical errors in 339 patients). These medical errors were categorized into nine types: communication problems (803 of2603), staff in caution (136 of 2603), lack of experience, knowledge or education (844 of 2603), lack of guidelines, protocols or policies (36 of 2603), intense work pressure (47 of 2603), staff deficiency (42 of 2603), poor awareness of staff (124 of 2603), environmental problems (226 of 2603), other issues (documentation issues, inadequate materials, poor organization, etc.) (345 of 2603), and employee or administration mistakes.

Medical errors were mainly encountered by 23.18 % in abdominal surgery, while they were encountered the least in cardiovascular surgery (10.03 %). This result provides a source of generalizable safety errors observed in the OR. The data were reviewed by the researches within practices, and medical errors in the integration of observations could exist. However, this study provides a rich source of information on the kinds of medical errors that are realized and the parameters that contribute to errors. Medical errors may have significant effects on patient safety and the quality of intra-operative care. Lack of experience, knowledge, oreducation and communication problems are the most common and significant priorities for the quality of intra-operative care. Literature reviews usually reported that patient safety was imperiled in the operating room due to broken communication, lack of information, and intense work pressure[9,10]. This study reviewed a series of unique situations of medical errors in intra-operative care in procedures with the main objective of learning from errors for the advantage of next patients. The data collected in this showed that the majority of medical errors that were identified were mainly caused by lack of healthcare professionals,their insufficient qualifications, and broken communication[11]. Some studies described issues in the patient safety culture in the OR. These results were in agreement with the findings of previous studies regardingthe patient safety culture dimension of problems in the OR by scores ranging from 30 % to 70 % across the performed surveys[10-13]. It is possible that medical errors found in intra-operative care are defined in other venues such as teamwork, effective communication, organizational learning, continuous improvement, and supervision. In our analysis, 30.84 % (621 of 2603) of the issues were communication-related. Moreover, in 31.96 % (832 of 2603) of the patients, diagnosis and intervention safety issues were identified by the researchers. These errors resulted in the need for additional procedures or treatments, including new practices. The results of this study offer a starting emphasis for revelation of the weaknesses of systems within the healthcare organization in the OR. The most common medical errors occur in the OR[14]. This is in agreement with the results of other studies. In addition to issues in communication and lack of information, there are other errors observed in intra-operative care such as transfer, diagnosis, aseptic interventions, specimen management, keep record phases, specimen collection, preservation, and transportation. The contributing parameters generally included mistakesrelated tobroken communication, information deficits, and teamwork. Intra-operative nurses should evaluate themselves and take action to prevent their identified medical errors.

Limitation

The study was realized as a single-center as a limitation principle.

Conclusion

The results of this study showed that medical errors in the operating room are common, but they are not diagnosed andnoticed, and these resultsreflectedthe universe. As there is a limited number of studies in this regard, this studyis an important source of information on the topic.

Based on the results, to minimize medical errors and achieve a higher quality of care, the following precautions may be proposed:

- raising awareness and knowledge of employees
- individuals' concentration acting more carefully
- improvement of direct preventive strategies by the management

Conflict of Interest

The authors declare that there is no conflict of interest regarding the publication of this article.

Funding

No funding was used in the study.

Acknowledgements

The authors would like to thank all of the participants and co-authors who participatedin this study.

References

1. Denver, CO. (2015). Guideline for Positioning the Patient. In: *Guidelines for Peri-Operative Practice*. AORN, Inc, 563–582.

2. SammerCE,LykensK,SinghKP,MainsD, &LackanNA. (2010). What Is Patient Safety Culture? A Review of the Literature. *J Nurs Scholarsh*, 42(2), 156–165.

3. Alfredsdottir, H., &Bjornsdottir, K. (2008). Nursing and Patient Safety in the Operating Room. *Journal of Advanced Nursing*, 61(1), 29–37. doi: 10.1111/j.1365-2648.2007.04462.x

4. KohnLT, CorriganJM, &DonaldsonMC, editors. (2000). *To Err Is Human: Building a Safer Health System*.Washington (DC): Committee on Quality of Health Care, Institute of Medicine, National Academy Press.

5. Gillespie, BM., &Marshall, A. (2015). Implementation of Safety Checklists in Surgery: ARealist Synthesis of Evidence. *BMC Surg Journal of Implementation Science*,10(137), 1–14.

6. AORN Recommended Practices Committee. (2001). Recommended Practices for Positioning the Patient in Te Peri-Operative Practice Setting. AORN J, 73, 231–238.

7. James, JT. (2013). A New, Evidence-Based Estimate of Patient Harms Associated with Hospital Care. *J Patient Saf*, 9, 122–128

8. Beuzekom, M., Boer, F.,Akerboom, &S., Hudson, P. (2013). Patient Safety in the Operating Room: An Intervention Study on Latent Risk Factors. *BMC Surg Journal of AORN*, 97(2), 274–279. doi: 10.1186/1471-2482-12-10

9. Griffin, FA., &Classen, DC. (2008). Detection of Adverse Events in Surgical Patients Using the Trigger Tool Approach. *Quality & Safety in Health Care*, 17, 25–38. doi:10.1136/qshc.2007.025080

10. Pimentel, MPT., Choi, S., Fiumara, K., Kachalia, A., &Urman, RD. (2017). Safety Culture in the Operating Room: Variability among Peri-Operative Healthcare Workers.*J Patient Saf*, 00:00–00 doi: 10.1097/ PTS.0000000000000385

11. UgurE,KaraS, YildirimS, &AkbalE. (2016). Medical Errors and Patient Safety in the Operating Room. *J Pak Med Assoc*. 66(5), 593–597. [PubMed: 27183943].

12. Mallouli, M., Tlili, MA., Aouicha, W., Ben Rejeb, M., Zedini, C., Salwa, A., …&Ajmi, T. (2017). Assessing Patient Safety Culture in Tunisian Operating Rooms: A Multicenter Study. *International Journal for Quality in Health Care*, 29(2), 176–182.

13. Carvalho, PA., Göttems, LBD., Pires, MRGM.,&Oliveira, MLCD. (2015). Safety Culture in the Operating Room of a Public Hospital in

the Perception of Health Care Professionals. *Revistalatino-americana de enfermagem*, 23(6), 1041–1048.

14. de VriesE, Ramrattan M, SmorenburgS, GoumaD, BoermeesterM. (2008). The Incidence and Nature of In-Hospital Adverse Events: ASystematic review. *Qual Saf Health Care*, 17:216–23.DOI: 10.1136/qshc.2007.023622.

Evin Korkmaz Turkurka[1], Fatma Eti Aslan[2], and Caferi Tayyar Selcuk[3]

Assessment of Pain Arising During Wound Dressing Change

Abstract: *Aim:* The aim of this study was to investigate the causes of pain arising during wound dressing change.

Methods: This study was a descriptive and correlational study. Our study evaluating the wound and dressing pain included 263 patients who agreed to participate. The patient and wound characteristics were analyzed using a form evaluating patients' sociodemographic characteristics. Of these patients, 250 who reported their pain were evaluated for wound pain and pain arising during wound dressing change.

Results: According to the age distribution of the patients, the youngest patient was 18 years old, the oldest patient was 97 years old. It was found that there were 56 patients with chronic disease. In terms of wound characteristics, it was found that 69.6 % of the patients had acute wound, serosanguinous and purulent structure according to exudate type was more common with 32.6 %. The wet-to-dry dressing change used as the dressing technique was the most commonly used technique. In terms of wound site, 41,5 % of the wounds were found to be in the upper limb. Of the patients with wound, 95.1 % (250) reported that they had pain due to wound. When we evaluated the pain severity during the dressing process, it was found that of the patients, 61.6 % (154) felt a mild pain before dressing, 32 % (80) felt a severe pain during wound dressing, and 44.4 % (111) felt a disturbing pain after dressing.

Conclusion: Based on the results of this study, it was found that the wrong choice of wound management and dressing were the causes of pain arising during dressing. In order to increase awareness, it is recommended that health workers participate in necessary trainings, care for the patient's demands, be in communication with the patient, reduce the level of stress, and exercise due care to minimize pain.

Keywords: Dressing Pain, Wound Pain, Assessment of Pain Arising During Dressing

Introduction

Wound is defined as the loss of normal integrity of the body, loss of anatomical structure, and function of the tissue by the physical damage of any agent (1,2).

Although there are various classifications for wound, they are divided into acute and chronic wounds depending on recovery period. An acute wound is a wound that occurs suddenly and does not leave any damage behind after healing. Whereas, a chronic wound is the disruption of skin integrity, an occurrence of functional loss. The healing process takes a long time in chronic wounds (3). Wound care is of great importance for wounds to heal. The goal of wound care is to protect the living tissue, to prevent further tissue destruction in the trauma- tized area and to prevent the development of infection, to accelerate the wound healing, to ensure the skin, and to revent the complications that may arise in other organs and systems (4). Wound care should be specific to patient. The type of wound, the health status of patient, the dressing technique used, the effec- tiveness of health professional applying dressing, the dressing material selected, and the precautions that are taken to protect the wound and surrounding tissues during wound dressing are important points to consider in wound healing and in affecting pain that will arise in wound care (5, 6).

The pain felt during the application and removal of dressing may increase patient's potential of noncompliance with treatment. Patients may avoid partici- pating in their clinical appointments or may delay dressing change if they do the care on their own (6). A good wound knowledge, good communication skills, multidisciplinary approach, carrying out the procedure gently without damaging the tissues have been indicated to be effective in reducing or relieving pain (7).

In the studies conducted, the conditions that triggered pain during wound dressing change have been found to be in contact of wound with air during the removal of dressing, cold solutions used for dressing, removal of dressing material attached to wound, maceration of wound and surrounding tissue, use of inappropriate wound care material, and debridement (7, 8). The pain arising during wound dressing and the stress caused by this pain have been reported to have negative effects on wound healing (9). Healthcare providers should min- imize the dressing pain and concern to keep the patient's health at the highest level (9).

Analgesics as well as non-pharmacological methods are used to reduce pain during wound dressing change. In a study, it was reported that the level of pain in 36 patients with a burn wound aged 8–57 years was decreased by the "virtual reality therapy" method (10). In another study, it was indicated that the virtual reality method used during the dressing of two soldiers wounded in the war had a significant reduction in the pain levels during the dressing of the patients (11). Although wound care products, treatment, and dressing techniques have been developed over the years, it is observed that it has not been paid enough attention to the holistic approach to pain and wound healing, and that the fact of dressing pain is still present (5).

Pain is the most undesired condition during wound dressing application. As in the case of dressing pain, taking measure in expected pain, not causing pain during the procedure, care, and dressing are among the main responsibilities of health professionals in our day. However, in the literature review, it was found that there was no recent comprehensive study on dressing pain.

Pain is caused by not performing the procedure gently during dressing, damaging the wound tissue while removing the dressing and not considering patient's complaints during dressing. Moreover, the cause of patient's wound and the meaning and importance given by patient to dressing may affect the perception of pain. Although this appears to be an expected problem, knowing the answers to the questions of how severe does the dressing procedure cause pain? Which type of wound is more painful? Do dressing materials and dressing techniques affect the severity of pain? contribute to taking measures to reduce the dressing pain.

Materials and Methods

The design of this study is descriptive, correlational. The universe of the study consisted of 752 patients admitted to the Plastic Surgery Outpatient Clinic of the University Hospital in Diyarbakir for dressing between February 5 and March 9, 2018. The study sample consisted of 263 patients aged 18 years and above and accepted to participate in the study. The data were collected by using the sociodemographic characteristics form and structured identification form. The data were analyzed in the form of wound characteristics, wound pain, and pain arising during dressing.

The SPSS Statistics V22.0 software package was used for statistical analyses while analyzing the data obtained from the study. Descriptive statistical methods (frequency, percentage, mean, standard deviation) were used while analyzing the study data. The Pearson's Chi-square test and the Fisher's Exact test were used to compare the categorical data. The results were evaluated at a confidence interval of 95 % and a significance level of $p < 0.05$.

Results

Sixty-five per cent (171) of the patients included in the study were male. In terms of the age distribution of the patients, 28.5 % (75) of the patients were found to be in the 20–29 age range. The percentage of the patients with chronic disease is 21.3 % (56 patients). In the analysis conducted according to the chronic disease type, it was found that 42.2 % (27) of the patients with chronic disease were found to have diabetes mellitus (DM). In terms of wound characteristics of the patients, it was determined that 69.6 % (183) of the patients had acute wound, 39.9 % (105) of the wound causes was surgery (surgical wound),

45.5 % (192) of the wound appearances were granulation tissue, 32.6 % (87) of the exudate types distributed as purulent-serosanguinous. In terms of the patient's "wound area (cm^2)" (62.670 ± 191.419), it was found that the smallest wound area was 2 cm^2, the largest wound area was 2400 cm^2; in terms of "the rate of burn wound (percentage)" (0.090 ± 0.120), it was found that the rate of smallest burn wound area was 1 % and the rate of largest burn wound area was 60 %. The burn degree for 94.6 % (53) of the patients with burn wound was found to be second degree. The wound of 41.5 % (118) of the patients was in the upper limb. It was determined that 95.1 % (250) of the patients with wound had wound-related pain. It was determined that of the patients, 43.3 % (239) felt pain during wound dressing change, 72.9 % (191) had pain due to wound, and 33.2 % (124) felt a throbbing pain. While evaluating the patient's pain during dressing, it was found that 28 % (175) of the patients felt more pain while cleaning the wound, 44.1 (153) of patients reported that short resting breaks during wound dressing reduced pain. It was determined that 53.6 % (134) of the patients did not use analgesic for their wound, and that 59.3 % (16) of the patients using analgesic used non-steroidal anti-inflammatory drugs. In the study, it was found that the sleep of 45.6 % (114) of the patients was affected from the wound pain. Of the patients, 67.6 % that the removal of dressing by being wetted during wound dressing reduced their pain. It was determined that, of the patients, 61.6 % (154) felt a mild pain before dressing, 32 % (80) felt a severe pain during wound dressing, and 44.4 % (111) felt a disturbing pain after dressing.

While assessing the patient's pain during wound dressing in Tab. 1, it is seen that of the patients, 28 % (175) felt more pain while cleaning the wound, 44.1 % (153) reported that short rest breaks during wound dressing reduced pain.

Only 34 patients answered the question of what are the approaches to reduce pain during dressing? Of the patients, 67.6 % (23) reported that removal of dressing by being wetted reduced their pain during dressing, as indicated in Tab. 2.

Discussion

Pain is an undesired and unpleasant feeling. However, many diseases and medical practices are painful. Among the medical practices and patient care procedures, dressing change is often painful. In the literature, a study by Szor et al. (1999) found that 87.5 % of the patients felt pain during wound dressing (12). Pursuant to the data obtained in this study, it was found that the rate of patients who felt pain due to wound was 95.1 %, and the rate of the patients

Tab. 1: Factors That Increase and Reduce The Pain Arising During Dressing

Factors that increase/reduce pain		*n	%**
Factors that increase pain (n=624)	Cleaning	175	28.0
	Applying wound dressing	164	26.3
	Removal of bandage	157	25.2
	Touching	128	20.5
	Total	624	100
Factors that reduce pain (n=347)	Short resting breaks	153	44.1
	Warm cleaning solutions	81	23.4
	Removing dressing on his/her own	73	21.0
	Analgesic drugs	40	11.5
	Total	347	100

* More than one answer was given.
** Percentage ratios were calculated according to the total number

Tab. 2: Approaches That Reduce Pain During Wound Dressing According to The Patients

Approaches that reduce pain	n*	%
Removal of dressing by being wetted	23	67.7
Gently treating of wound tissue	6	17.7
Analgesic use	3	8.8
Short Breaks	1	2.9
Distraction while dressing	1	2.9
Total	34	100

* Only 34 of the patients answered this question

who felt pain during wound dressing from these patients was 49.1 %. In the literature, the study conducted by Bowers et al. (2009) determined that the conditions triggering pain during wound dressing change were contact of wound with air during the removal of dressing, cold solutions used for dressing, removal of dressing material attached to wound, maceration of wound and surrounding tissue, use of inappropriate wound care material and debridement (7). In the literature, the study conducted by Jones in 2017 reported that one of the most important causes of pain arising during wound dressing was the selection of inappropriate dressing material (13). In the literature, the study by Edwars conducted in 2011 reported that pain during wound dressing may sometimes be more severe than wound pain, and factors causing this pain were the removal of adhesive dressing and inadequate exudation management. The wound should be well known and wound-specific care should be given while applying dressing (14). Considering the wounds of the patients within the scope of our study, it was determined that 69.6 % (183) of the patients had acute wound according the time of wound formation, 39.9 % (105) of the wound causes was surgery (surgical wound), 45.5 % (192) of the wound appearances were granulation tissue, 32.6 % (87) of the exudate types distributed as purulent-serosanguinous. In this study, it was found that wet-to-dry dressing was applied with a rate of 82.5 % (217 patients) as the characteristic of dressing used. It was determined that 28 % of the factors increasing the dressing pain occurred during the cleaning of wound site, and that taking short rest breaks during wound dressing was effective in 44.1 % of the pain-relieving factors. In the literature, a study by Szor et al. conducted in 1999 reported that 18 % of the patients described their pain arising during wound dressing change as "terrible" or "excruciating" (12). In our study, it was determined that of the patients, 61.6 % (154) felt a mild pain before dressing, 32 % (80) felt a severe pain during wound dressing, and 44.4 % (111) felt a disturbing pain after dressing. In the literature, the study by Szor et al. in 1999 reported that analgesic was prescribed to only 6 % of the patients to relieve their pain, although pain was felt during wound dressing (12). In this study, it was determined that 53.6 % (134) of the patients did not use analgesic for their wound, and that 59.3 % (16) of the patients using analgesic used non-steroidal anti-inflammatory drugs. In our study, 34 patients gave various recommendations for pain relief during dressing. Of these, 67.7 % asked that the dressing be removed by being wetted, 17.7 % asked that the wound tissue be treated delicately, 8.8 % asked that analgesic be applied, 2.9 % asked to be distracted during dressing.

Wounds are often painful. In the literature, the study by Kim et al. conducted in 2016 reported that another cause of pain arising during wound dressing was skin irritations and tears as a result of dressing removal, which was mostly caused by frequent dressing changes in chronic wounds such as pressure sores (5). It was indicated that skin irritations and tears may cause new wounds, as well as enlarging the wound size and increasing the pain. The pain severity of wounds varies depending on the structure, size, and characteristics of wound. Considering the size of wounds that we evaluated in our study, it was determined that the smallest wound area (cm^2) was 2 cm^2 and the largest wound area was 2400 cm^2, and in terms of "the rate of burn wound (percentage)", it was determined that the rate of smallest burn wound area was 1 % and the rate of largest burn wound area was 60 %. It was found that the dressing of burn wound, one of the painful dressing procedures, increased the duration and severity of pain depending on the size of wound site. In the literature, a study by Feber et al. conducted in 2013 reported that the virtual reality method used to reduce the pain level of patients during wound dressing was effective (10). In this study, 2.9 % of 34 patients, who answered the question of "Was there any factor that relieved your pain during dressing?, reported that distraction reduced their pain. Considering the literature and the results of our study, it was observed that most of the wounds were painful and the wound structure, presence of infection, frequency of dressing, and approach to the patient were effective on pain severity.

A wound-specific care is required to reduce the pain arising during dressing. It was found that of the dressing techniques used in our study, 82.5 % were wet-to-dry dressing, 13.3 % were dry dressing, 3.8 % were negative-pressure dressing, and 0.4 % were synthetic dressing. In the literature, the study conducted by Yıldırım et al. in 2012 showed that the dry dressing technique used for intensely draining wounds caused pain during the removal of dressing because of the high probability of infection as the site is more permeable to air and adherence to the wound exudate (15). In our study, 25.2 % of the patients reported that their pain increased when the dressing bandage was removed. Twenty-one per cent of the patients reported that their pain reduced when they removed the dressings themselves. It was observed that 23 of the patients asked the dressing bandage to be wetted with saline solution before removal. In the literature, the study conducted by Ayhan et al. (2009) reported that negative-pressure dressing techniques decreased pain compared with other techniques (16). In this study, the negative-pressure dressing technique was used for ten patients. One of these patients reported no pain in the wound. Of the nine patients who reported pain during wound dressing, five indicated that the pain was very severe during wound dressing and four reported that their pain was unbearable. Our study is not consistent with the literature. The reason for this is due to the fact that the healthcare professionals who used the negative-pressure dressing technique lacked knowledge on using the technique or did not receive adequate training. Considering the material aspect of the dressing techniques used, the choice of appropriate technique for patient comfort and to shorten the healing period instead of using the cheap technique should be the primary responsibility of the person applying the dressing.

The literature and the results of this study show that most of the patients experience pain during dressing, suggesting ethical violations in care. Because the principle of "first, do no harm" (Premium non nocera) in health care is one of the basic principles that should be kept in mind.

Conclusion

The results obtained from this study were found to be as follows: the causes of pain experienced by patients during wound dressing were due to the lack of knowledge on wound, incorrect wound management, selection of wrong dressing technique, not treating the tissues gently because of not sharing enough time to the patient, prolonged healing process and frequent dressing application caused by not performing wound debridement, delaying the wound care since the patient feel pain during wound dressing, resulting in worsened wound exudate. It was also found that the patient's inadequate personal hygiene caused delay of the wound healing, resulting in exposure to frequent painful dressing procedures.

Based on these results, it is recommended that

Healthcare personnel providing wound care should participate in required courses and certificate programs to specialize in wound care,

The institution policy follow the innovations in wound care and meet the required lacking material to provide proper care to the patient by considering the patient's comfort and shortening of the healing process,

Healthcare personnel applying dressing help minimize dressing pain by considering patient's demands,

To give short rest breaks during wound dressing procedure to reduce the dressing pain of the patients, to distract the patient and to evaluate the effectiveness of this method by using music or various alternative methods.

References

1. Tepebasi, M.Y., and Calapoglu, N.S., 2016. Cellular and molecular mechanism of wound healing. *Medical Journal of Suleyman Demirel University.* **23** (4), pp. 140–146.

2. Parsak, C.K., Sakman, G. and Celik, U., 2007. Wound healing, wound care and complications. *Archives Medical Review Journal.* **16** (2), pp. 145–159.

3. Cakır Umar, D. and Turhan Damar, H., 2017. Acute and Chronic Wounds and Nursing care. *Turkish Journal of Clinics.* **3** (3), pp. 157–163.

4. Akyuz, N., 2008. Basic principles of wound healing and care. *Istanbul University Cerrahpasa Faculty of Medicine Continuing Medical Education Activities Symposium Series.* **67**, pp. 11–15.

5. Kim, J.Y., Kim, N.K. and Lee, Y.L., 2016. A descriptive study of korean nurses' perception of pain and skin tearing at dressing change. *International Wound Journal.* **13**, pp. 47–51.

6. Ross, G.S., 2004. Surgical wound care: current views on minimising dressing-related pain. *Manchester Royal Infirmary.* **20** (1), pp. 38–40.

7. Bowers, K. and Barrett, S., 2009. Wound-related pain: features, assessment and treatment. *Continuing Professional Development, Primary Health Care.* **19**, pp. 37–45.

8. Upton, D. and Solowiej, K., 2010. Pain and stress as contributors to delayed wound healing. *Wound Practice and Research.* **3**, pp. 114–122.

9. Upton, D., 2014. Psychological aspects of wound care: implications for clinical practice *Wound Care JCN.* **28**(2), pp. 52–57.

10. Feber, A.W., Patterson, D.R. and Bremer, M., 2013. Repeated use of immersive virtual reality therapy to control pain during wound dressing changes in pediatric and adult burn patients. *National Institutes of Health Public Access.* **34** (4), pp. 563–568.

11. Maani, C., Hoffman, H.G., Desocio, P.A., Morrow, M., Galin, C., Magula, J., Maiers, A. and Gaylord, K., 2008. Pain control during wound care for combat-related burn injuries using custom articulated arm mounted virtual reality goggles. *Journal of Cybertherapy and Rehabilitation.* **1** (2), pp. 193–198.

12. Szor, J.K. and Bourguignon, C., 1999. Description of pressure ulcer pain at rest and at dressing change. *Journal of WOCN.* **26** (3), pp. 115–120.

13. Jones, J. and Williams, H., 2017. Wound management should not be a pain. *British Journal of Community Nursing.* **22** (9), pp. 38–46.

14. Edwards, J., 2011. Managing wound pain in patients with burns using soft silicone dressings. *Wounds UK.* **7** (4), pp. 122–126.

15. Yildirim, A.O., Tuncer, S.K., Bayram, Y., Eyi, Y.E., Eroglu, M. and Ozenc, S., 2012. Use of wound care products in the emergency department. *TAF Preventive Medicine Bulletin.* **11** (6), pp. 773–778.

16. Ayhan, H., Sahin, I., Tastan, S., Bilgen, E. and Hatioglu, S., 2009. Healthcare providers' views on the use of vacuum-assisted closure and modern dressings in wound care. *Turkish Journal of Plastic Reconstructive and Aesthetic Surgery.* **17** (1), pp. 11–15.

Gökay Kurtulan

Hospital Disaster Plan in Istanbul Hospitals: Evaluation from a Strategic Planning Perspective

Abstract: Objective: The aim of this research was to examine the disaster planning processes (including before and after period of the preparation of the disaster plan) and to determine the current situation.

Material and Method: In order to evaluate the critical facilities and capabilities of the hospitals before, during and after the preparation of the disaster plan, a Likert-type scale which including strategic planning principles was used and hospitals were classified according to their scores. All hospitals within the provincial borders of Istanbul were accepted as a universe and sample was not taken.

Results: A total of 146 (71 % of the universe) hospitals, 52 of them were state, 7 of them were university and 87 of them were private; and it was determined that 87 % of hospitals had Hospital Disaster Plan (HDP). According to the scoring, disaster planning was found at a good level in 40.9 % of the hospitals which have disaster plan, moderate in 43.3 % of the hospitals and 15.8 % of them were found inadequate in disaster planning.

Conclusion: The preparation of the written documents of the disaster plan does not mean that hospitals are ready for disasters. Hospitals need to complete other disaster-related preparations additionally written documents. Using strategic planning as a basic tool in the preparation of disaster preparedness allows hospitals to base their activities on concrete work programs and budgets and to monitor and evaluate their practices effectively. The units in which the representatives of different disciplines are required to control, measure, evaluate and certify the disaster preparedness levels of hospitals based on the standard criteria to be determined are needed.

Keywords: Disaster Preparedness, Hospital Disaster Plan Hospital Incident Management System, Hospital Incident Command System, Strategic Disaster Planning

Introduction

It has been proven that if societies are unprepared for unusual situations, the negativity will have a greater impact. This is also valid for the hospitals. Of course, hospitals are structures that are not exempt from the catastrophic effects of disaster in possible disasters. Preparing plans for disasters, testing and continual updating of these plans can eliminate or mitigate the negative impact of problems (1,2).

Hospitals have a complex structure within their service areas and size. There is a need for a system where effective and common language is spoken in order to be able to intervene in the shortest and most effective way in the event of an incident, to continue the operation in the event and after the event and to provide the best service (3).

Hospitals have always high probability of being affected by disasters. Because they are complex structures, host intensive people for 24 hours a day contain critical materials and hazardous substances within their body, have heavy medical equipment and supplies and hospitals are the basic facilities that always need energy resources (4). Past disasters have shown us that it is inevitable for the hospital to be affected by the fire, explosion, building collapse, faults in the water network, spread of infection and similar events in the hospital. In addition, the storm, drought, flood, avalanche, landslide, earthquake, volcanic eruption, major accidents, explosions, fire, building, dam, tunnel collapse, such as poisoning of water and food, terror and similar events outside the hospital can affect the hospital directly or indirectly. In these cases, the hospital may be directly subject to disasters and damaged or may apply to the position to those who are exposed to disaster. In short, there may be cases where both the hospital is affected and has become the applicant (5).

In the early times of a disaster, chaos is inevitable. The goal should be reduced this time to the least possible time (6). In the event of any disaster, the most common and most service-expected facilities will be the hospitals. Hospitals are required to complete disaster preparedness in order to survive all kinds of disasters and continue to provide uninterrupted service. It is also determined that the importance of disaster management is not given in most of the hospitals located within the borders of Istanbul Metropolitan Municipality (7).

Planning is the first and most important stage of management work as well as management activity begins with planning. The plan is to decide today, where to reach in the future and what is desired to be realized (8). The answers to those questions "Where are we?", "Where do we want to reach?", "How to reach where we want to go?" and "How we follow and evaluate our success?" constitute the strategic planning process of an organization (9).

Hospital disaster plan is a struggle system against to disaster. This system comes into play immediately during a disaster and approaches the event in a systematic way. The tasks of the people involved are well planned and defined in advance. Hospital disaster plan prepares the organization and its employees for disasters before disaster. Hospital disaster plan requires regular keeping of records. A common and comprehensible language should be used to ensure that the plan is understood in the same way by all concerned (10).

The purpose of the hospital disaster plan is being successful and organized in the diagnosis and treatment of the patients who sent to hospital after a disaster, to minimize the problems that may occur by preventing panic and confusion within the hospital due to disaster, to determine the responsible person and duties of each unit in this plan in advance and to provide a good organization among the units (11).

Hospital disaster plans should be prepared without waiting for disaster. Each hospital should prepare a special disaster plan. Because the physical structure of each hospital, economic conditions, the number of personnel and the distribution of the personnel among the branches, the geographic area where it is located and the socio-cultural structure of the environment are not the same (2).

Materials and Methods

This research is a descriptive study conducted to evaluate the current state of disaster plans of hospitals within the provincial borders of Istanbul. The universe of the study consists of the hospitals within the provincial borders of Istanbul. For this purpose, according to the hospital list provided by Istanbul Provincial Health Directorate, a total of 206 hospitals, 52 of them are state, 7 of them are universities and 147 of them are private, are designated as the universe of the research. The sampling was not carried out and it was aimed to include all hospitals in the research.

A literature review was performed for data collection tool and a scale was developed to answer the research questions. Developed scale consists of 3 parts.

- In the first chapter, there are 4 questions about whether the hospital has a disaster plan, the reasons for not having a disaster plan and whether the preparation of disaster plan is foreseen in the forthcoming period.
- In the second part, there are 5 questions about the duty of participant, whether they have been involved in the disaster plan preparation, whether they have received training on disaster planning, the number of beds in the hospital and how the disaster plan is named in the hospital.
- The third and the last part of the research used as a scale, there are 89 points to be scored with 1–5 score points. These are:
  - 12 statements regarding the activities of hospitals before the disaster plan was prepared.
  - 49 statements related to the activities of hospitals in the preparation of disaster plan.

- 6 statements regarding the activities of hospitals after the disaster plan was prepared.
- 22 statements regarding the critical facilities and capabilities that hospitals will use or need to use in a disaster.

The data were collected through face-to-face interviews and Marmara University internet survey system. Necessary permits were obtained from the relevant official institutions for the participation of state and university hospitals in the research. Private Hospitals and Health Institutions Association was supported to inform private hospitals about the research and to participate in the research. Research data, if any, from each hospital's disaster planning responsible; otherwise, it is ensured that the most qualified personnel (Chief Physician, Assistant Chief Physician, Hospital Manager, etc.) are assigned to respond on behalf of the hospital. 71 % of 206 hospitals that form the universe participated in this research.

The alpha coefficient (Cronbach Alpha) was used to test the reliability of the scale used in the study. Data obtained from 146 hospitals were used in the analysis. In addition, in order to determine how and what extent the expressions affect the alpha coefficient; "Alpha if Item Deleted" value is calculated. These values indicate the internal consistency of the remaining variables if any variable is deleted. As a result of the internal consistency of the 89-item scale for the study, a high reliability level of $\alpha = 0.976$ was obtained (Tabs. 1–4).

Tab. 1: The Effects of the Substances Forming the Period Before the Preparation of the Disaster Plan on the Reliability

Item	Mean	S.D.	Scale Average When Item Deleted	Scale Variance When Item Deleted	Corrected Matter All Correlation	Item Deleted Cronbach Alpha
c3before	4,11	0,96	39,449	105,821	0,612	0,922
c4before	4,13	0,97	39,433	104,470	0,680	0,920
c5before	3,93	1,24	39,630	99,108	0,736	0,917
c6before	3,70	1,26	39,858	98,440	0,752	0,916
c7before	3,57	1,21	39,992	97,865	0,814	0,914
c8before	3,97	1,15	39,591	99,561	0,785	0,915
c9before	4,03	1,08	39,528	100,759	0,778	0,916
c10before	3,54	1,40	40,024	100,245	0,593	0,924
c11before	3,57	1,19	39,992	100,833	0,693	0,919
c12before	2,68	1,44	40,882	101,375	0,533	0,927
c13before	3,20	1,34	40,362	99,423	0,660	0,920
c14before	3,15	1,36	40,409	98,656	0,681	0,919

Tab. 2: The Effects of the Substances Forming the Period Factor on the Reliability of the Preparation Process of the Disaster Plan

Item	Mean	S.D.	Scale Average When Item Deleted	Scale Variance When Item Deleted	Corrected Matter All Correlation	Item Deleted Cronbach Alpha
c15process	3,795	1,335	153,937	1570,123	0,533	0,968
c16process	4,102	1,007	153,630	1576,933	0,630	0,968
c17process	4,126	1,062	153,606	1576,558	0,601	0,968
c18process	3,535	1,153	154,197	1570,763	0,615	0,968
c19process	2,953	1,419	154,780	1554,411	0,642	0,968
c20process	2,409	1,353	155,323	1579,839	0,434	0,968
c21process	3,433	1,429	154,299	1550,180	0,676	0,967
c22process	3,362	1,349	154,370	1554,933	0,673	0,967
c23process	2,811	1,332	154,921	1558,645	0,646	0,968
c24process	3,244	1,344	154,488	1554,966	0,675	0,967
c25process	2,748	1,464	154,984	1554,158	0,624	0,968
c26process	2,811	1,283	154,921	1562,438	0,633	0,968
c27process	2,575	1,616	155,157	1554,467	0,559	0,968
c28process	2,551	1,384	155,181	1552,245	0,680	0,967
c29process	3,268	1,281	154,465	1555,695	0,702	0,967
c30process	3,575	1,199	154,157	1558,816	0,719	0,967
c31process	3,488	1,161	154,244	1558,122	0,751	0,967
c32process	3,661	1,093	154,071	1561,352	0,762	0,967
c33process	3,394	1,304	154,339	1559,130	0,655	0,968
c34process	3,638	1,186	154,094	1559,134	0,723	0,967
c35process	3,732	1,144	154,000	1570,302	0,625	0,968
c36process	3,512	1,188	154,220	1557,729	0,738	0,967
c37process	3,071	1,304	154,661	1563,924	0,608	0,968
c38process	3,118	1,707	154,614	1582,461	0,316	0,969
c39process	2,181	1,477	155,551	1569,726	0,482	0,968
c40process	2,268	1,422	155,465	1565,790	0,537	0,968
c41process	3,165	1,703	154,567	1560,136	0,485	0,968
c42process	2,882	1,703	154,850	1555,557	0,520	0,968
c43process	3,976	1,275	153,756	1566,249	0,599	0,968
c44process	4,165	1,160	153,567	1572,755	0,589	0,968
c45process	4,197	1,182	153,535	1575,457	0,548	0,968
c46process	4,339	1,033	153,394	1586,622	0,494	0,968
c47process	4,220	1,083	153,512	1578,426	0,566	0,968

(continued on next page)

Tab. 2: (continued)

Item	Mean	S.D.	Scale Average When Item Deleted	Scale Variance When Item Deleted	Corrected Matter All Correlation	Item Deleted Cronbach Alpha
c48process	3,409	1,422	154,323	1550,649	0,675	0,967
c49process	2,921	1,592	154,811	1552,789	0,582	0,968
c50process	3,669	1,517	154,063	1553,869	0,603	0,968
c51process	4,386	1,016	153,346	1590,339	0,456	0,968
c52process	3,575	1,400	154,157	1553,673	0,658	0,968
c53process	3,953	1,441	153,780	1566,491	0,524	0,968
c54process	3,315	1,401	154,417	1537,372	0,810	0,967
c55process	3,213	1,349	154,520	1537,712	0,839	0,967
c56process	3,071	1,352	154,661	1539,638	0,818	0,967
c57process	2,614	1,316	155,118	1547,359	0,765	0,967
c58process	2,835	1,356	154,898	1540,855	0,805	0,967
c59process	2,945	1,399	154,787	1533,931	0,843	0,967
c60process	3,945	1,405	153,787	1570,248	0,504	0,968
c61process	3,575	1,591	154,157	1556,023	0,556	0,968
c62process	3,575	1,591	154,157	1556,023	0,556	0,968
c63process	3,575	1,591	154,157	1556,023	0,556	0,968

Tab. 3: The Effects of the Substances Forming the Period Factor on the Reliability after the Preparation of the Disaster Plan

Item	Mean	S.D.	Scale Average When Item Deleted	Scale Variance When Item Deleted	Corrected Matter All Correlation	Item Deleted Cronbach Alpha
c65after	3,252	1,363	16,173	37,081	0,876	0,913
c66after	3,016	1,409	16,409	37,339	0,822	0,920
c67after	3,197	1,375	16,228	36,495	0,908	0,909
c68after	2,898	1,391	16,528	36,807	0,873	0,913
c69after	3,827	1,369	15,598	40,036	0,667	0,939
c70after	3,236	1,519	16,189	37,964	0,705	0,936

While evaluating the findings obtained in the study, NCSS & PASS Statistical Software (Utah, USA) program was used for statistical analysis. In addition to descriptive statistical methods (mean, standard deviation), the conformity of the parameters to normal distribution was evaluated with Kolmogorov-Smirnov test.

Tab. 4: The Effects of Substances That Constitute the Facility and Capability Factor on Reliability

Item	Mean	S.D.	Scale Average When Item Deleted	Scale Variance When Item Deleted	Corrected Matter All Correlation	Item Deleted Cronbach Alpha
c71faccap	3,863	1,218	67,466	277,671	0,404	0,869
c72faccap	3,945	1,131	67,384	277,286	0,451	0,868
c73faccap	2,842	1,579	68,486	268,652	0,472	0,867
c74faccap	3,733	1,454	67,596	271,994	0,448	0,868
c75faccap	3,788	1,350	67,541	273,450	0,455	0,868
c76faccap	4,027	1,197	67,301	286,143	0,197	0,874
c77faccap	2,685	1,489	68,644	274,424	0,384	0,870
c78faccap	3,596	1,367	67,733	270,128	0,524	0,866
c79faccap	3,623	1,518	67,705	272,140	0,422	0,869
c80faccap	2,692	1,672	68,637	268,233	0,448	0,868
c81faccap	2,342	1,524	68,986	271,227	0,439	0,868
c82faccap	2,356	1,475	68,973	270,372	0,475	0,867
c83faccap	3,253	1,457	68,075	267,215	0,551	0,865
c84faccap	2,253	1,457	69,075	266,222	0,573	0,864
c85faccap	2,945	1,685	68,384	260,776	0,587	0,863
c86faccap	3,281	1,713	68,048	262,225	0,548	0,864
c87faccap	2,500	1,707	68,829	276,570	0,283	0,874
c88faccap	2,740	1,710	68,589	266,782	0,463	0,868
c89faccap	3,171	1,699	68,158	257,913	0,637	0,861
c90faccap	4,089	1,481	67,240	272,515	0,427	0,869
c91faccap	4,308	1,306	67,021	279,455	0,330	0,871
c92faccap	3,295	1,523	68,034	269,357	0,478	0,867

The One Way Anova test was used to compare normal distribution parameters according to groups of three or more. Tukey HSD test was used to determine the group that caused the difference. Student t-test was used in the evaluation according to two groups. Kruskal Wallis test was used to compare the parameters that did not show normal distribution. The Mann Whitney U test was used to determine the difference between these two groups. Chi-square test was used to compare qualitative datas. Validity analyzes were evaluated with Cronbach Alpha coefficient. The results were evaluated at 95 %, confidence interval and $p < 0.05$ at significance level.

Tab. 5: Classification of Hospitals According to Ratings (13,14)

Classification of the hospital	Point
C Class Hospital	0–35
B Class Hospital	36–65
A Class Hospital	>65

In the last section of the data collection tool, 89 expressions were scored within 1–5 score points. Six different points were calculated by using the points obtained as a result of the scoring. These are: "HDP BEFORE Point", "HDP PROCESS Point", "HDP AFTER Point", "HDP Point", "FACCAP Point" and "GENERAL Point". In the calculation of points, for all items in one dimension, score points 1 to 5 are collected. First, this total was multiplied by 100, then divided by the number of items and the number multiplied by 5. The resulting number, multiplied by 1.25 and 25 value was subtracted from the result. Thus a score out of 100 was obtained (12).

After the scoring, hospitals are classified into 3 categories as shown in Tab. 5, based on the "Hospital Safety Index Guide for Evaluators" prepared by the Pan American Health Organization Regional Office of the World Health Organization as a hospital evaluation document (13,14).

Results

87 % of the hospitals that collected data stated that they had a disaster plan; however, 13 % did not (Tab. 6).

When HDP points of 127 hospitals, which have a disaster plan are examined, it has been calculated that 17,3 % of them between 0–35, 41 % of them between 36–65 and 41,7 % of them above 65. When GENERAL points of the same hospitals are analyzed, it has been calculated that 15,8 % of them between 0–35, 43,3 % of them between 36–65 and 40,9 % of them above 65 (Table 7).

There was a statistically significant rise (p <0.05) in HDP BEFORE, HDP PROCESS, HDP AFTER and HDP points of non Education and Research State Hospitals (ERH). There is no statistically significant difference between FACCAP and GENERAL points of public hospitals according to being ERH (p>0,05). While the rate of ERH is high among state hospitals with HDP score between 0–35, there is a high rate of non-ERH among state hospitals with more than 65 HDP points (p<0,05) (Tab. 8 and 9).

Tab. 6: Distribution of Hospitals According to Having Disaster Plan

Hospital Disaster Plan	n	%
There is	127	87
There is not	19	13
TOTAL	146	100

Tab. 7: Distribution of HDP and GENERAL Scores of Hospitals Has Disaster Plan.

Point		n	%
HDP Point	0–35 (C)	22	17,3
	36–65 (B)	52	41,0
	> 65 (A)	53	41,7
GENERAL Point	0–35 (C)	20	15,8
	36–65 (B)	55	43,3
	> 65 (A)	52	40,9

Tab. 8: Distribution of HDP and GENERAL Scores of State Hospitals According to Being ERH

Point		ERH		Not ERH	
		n	%	n	%
HDP Point	0-35 (C)	8	34,8	2	8,3
	36-65 (B)	10	43,5	9	37,5
	> 65 (A)	5	21,7	13	54,2
GENERAL Point	0-35 (C)	7	30,4	2	8,3
	36-65 (B)	10	43,5	10	41,7
	> 65 (A)	6	26,1	12	50,0

There was a statistically significant rise ($p < 0,01$) in HDP BEFORE, HDP PROCESS, HDP AFTER, HDP, FACCAP and GENERAL points of hospitals that have JCI accreditation. The rate of having JCI accreditation is high in the hospitals that have HDP and GENERAL points more than 65 (Tab. 10 and 11).

Tab. 9: Evaluation of the Scores of State Hospitals According to Being an ERH

Point		ERH		Not ERH		p
		Mean±SD (Median)		Mean±SD (Median)		
HDP Before Point		49,96±26,76		67,36±19,29		*0,014**
HDP Process Point		48,13±23,14		61,58±18,31		*0,032**
+HDP After Point		44,56±28,61 (45,83)		61,81±25,99 (62,5)		*0,027**
HDP Point		48,15±23,43		62,64±18,16		*0,022**
FACCAP Point		51,57±19,55		51,01±16,06		*0,909*
GENARAL Point		49,14±21,61		60,03±15,85		*0,054*
		n	%	n	%	
++HDP Point	0-35 (C)	8	34,8	2	8,3	*0,027**
	36-65 (B)	10	43,5	9	37,5	
	> 65 (A)	5	21,7	13	54,2	
++GENERAL Point	0-35 (C)	7	30,4	2	8,3	*0,093*
	36-65 (B)	10	43,5	10	41,7	
	> 65 (A)	6	26,1	12	50,0	

Student t test was used
+Mann-Whitney U test
++Ki-Kare test
*p<0,05

Tab. 10: Distribution of HDP and GENERAL Scores According to Having JCI Accreditation

Point		Has JCI Accreditation		Has not JCI Accreditation	
		n	%	n	%
HDP Point	0-35 (C)	-	-	22	20,4
	36-65 (B)	5	26,3	47	43,5
	> 65 (A)	14	73,7	39	36,1
GENERAL Point	0-35 (C)	-	-	20	18,5
	36-65 (B)	4	21,1	51	47,2
	> 65 (A)	15	78,9	37	34,3

Tab. 11: Evaluation of Scores According to JCI Accreditation Status

Point		Has JCI Accreditation Mean±SD (Median)		Has Not JCI Accreditation Mean±SD (Median)		p
HDP Before Point		78,94±17,93		63,42±22,73		*0,006***
HDP Process Point		76,63±15,19		54,88±20,81		*0,001***
+HDP After Point		88,37±15,50 (100)		50,23±28,86 (50)		*0,001***
HDP Point		78,10±15,31		55,99±20,42		*0,001***
FACCAP Point		78,64±12,04		52,67±18,16		*0,001***
GENARAL Point		78,23±13,94		55,28±18,62		*0,001***
		n	**%**	**n**	**%**	
++HDP Point	*0-35 (C)*	-	-	22	20,4	*0,005***
	36-65 (B)	5	26,3	47	43,5	
	> 65 (A)	14	73,7	39	36,1	
++GENERAL Point	*0-35 (C)*	-		20	18,5	*0,001***
	36-65 (B)	4	21,1	51	47,2	
	> 65 (A)	15	78,9	37	34,3	

Student t test was used
+Mann-Whitney U test
++Ki-Kare test

Discussion

Research data, if any, gathered from each hospital's custodian for disaster planning, otherwise, it is gathered from its authorized staff to respond on behalf of the hospital. It was determined that two-thirds of the hospitals were responsible for the planning of the disaster and the staff of the head and their assistants, the hospital director and his assistants and one-third of the staff in the other positions. It has been found that in state hospitals, Assistant Chief Physicians have been assigned in general, but disaster planning is carried out under the responsibility of "other personnel" in private hospitals. In the distribution of other personnel are head nurse, civil defense expert, quality manager, administrative personnel, training officer, operation staff, general coordinator, etc. There were many different areas of staff who work in different areas. This situation shows that the planning of disaster is not precisely determined by who or which departments should be carried out in hospitals. It would be most appropriate method to carry out disaster planning under the responsibility of a team composed of different disciplines.

It has been determined that the majority of the participant staff who are responsible for disaster planning has received training on the disaster plan. However, a considerable part of those was not trained. In the majority of hospitals, the requirement for training in the period prior to the preparation of the disaster plan has not been determined exactly and it has been determined that the training on hospital disaster planning has not been implicitly taken during the plan preparation period. Bozkırlı (2004) states in his research which consists of 31 hospitals in Ankara that 67,8 % of hospital representatives who participated this study did not receive hospital disaster planning training (15). Bartley, Stella and Walsh (2006), 50 of a hospital's senior 170 staff likely to be critical in the event of a disaster; first a pre-test with 50 questions followed by a 1-hour simulated disaster lecture and finally a post-test with 42 questions. There was a significant difference between pre-test and post-test in favor of development. In the pre-test, 18 % of the staff was successful, while 50 % of the staff was successful in the final test. In the study, the information levels of the emergency services employees were higher than the others. As a result of the study, it has been shown that disaster drills and training process provide direct benefits to both personnel and staff working in the same way, as well as similar practices has contributed to the development of disaster plans. In order to increase the disaster preparedness of hospitals, it is emphasized that training and demonstration activities should be done more (16). As a result of the research conducted by Sarp and İşlek (2006), in order to determine the level of knowledge of a hospital staff on fire, it was determined that a significant number of the respondents had misunderstood or did not know how to behave in the event of a fire, most of them had misinformation about the fire precautions, teams and equipment in the hospital or had no information. It was also determined that only 12.4 % of the participants were trained about fire and the hospital did not perform any demonstration or training about fire (17). It should be compulsory for hospitals to be trained in disaster planning without public and private discrimination. It is required that the personnel who will give training will be required to have graduate education in hospital disaster planning and/or to participate in domestic/foreign courses. Authorization of the Ministry of Health shall be appropriate for individuals and institutions that will provide education.

It was reported that only one third of the hospital buildings were exactly resistant to serious earthquakes. This situation is considered to be a big problem for Istanbul where it has a serious earthquake risk. Disaster status of the health institutions expected to serve in the event of a disaster will adversely affect the health services after the earthquake and will lead to inability to use the resources. Paul and Lin (2009) stated that any structural and non-structural damage may occur in hospitals after disasters will weaken the capabilities of hospitals (18). Istanbul Metropolitan Municipality Planning and Development Department Ground and Earthquake Inspection Directorate (2003) recommends the investigation of the microarea and geological and physical features of the hospitals (risk status of the floor where hospitals are located, distances to faults and possible effects etc.) in order to determine the risks for determining and reducing the positional risks of hospitals. Additionally, in order to reduce the structural risks after the risks are determined, it is recommended that the durability of the hospital structure should be determined, the ones that need improvement, the determination of the standards within the structure and the development of intervention forms for structural risks (19).

Nearly half of the hospitals have been able to meet their own electricity, water, medical gas and nutritional needs for at least 3 days in the condition of deduction or no replenishing. This situation shows that half of the hospitals may become inoperable after a disaster has occurred. Bozkırlı (2004), in his research on 31 hospitals in Ankara, found that 58 % of the hospitals had spare generators and 67.7 % of them had spare water tanks (15). In general, American College of Emergency Physicians, Federal Emergency Management Agency (FEMA) (2005) states that hospitals should be able to meet their own electricity, fuel, medical gas and catering needs for at least 3 days without any help and that alternative water sources other than main water should be available (20). In Turkey, this duration (at least 3 days) should be approved as a standard and hospitals should be applied as an essential requirement in the licensing process.

It is determined that if some of the hospitals become partially or completely unavailable after the disaster, there is no space for the hospital to set up as a mobile and there are no tents and equipment to set up the hospital; there is no separate decontamination and triage area of the hospitals except for the emergency department; personnel had no personal protective equipment; there were no equipment and medical equipment needed to intervene in cases of radioactive material victims; there is no automatic telephone or message system which can call the hospital staff and there is no radio system, fire detection system and fire escape. This situation shows that some of the hospitals will have difficulties in providing services after the disaster and managerial problems will come into prominence. It may be normal for hospitals to have differences in some possibilities and capabilities. However, it is necessary to set minimum standards for the facilities and capabilities that will be needed after the disaster.

It was determined that decontamination procedures could not be performed in one third of hospitals. In an environment where the risk of terror is always present, hospitals should primarily protect their own staff and prevent their hospitals from being contaminated. This condition shows that most of our hospitals are not fully prepared for patients who will need decontamination. Kaji and Lewis (2006), in their research on 45 hospitals, found that 51 % of the hospitals had chemical antidote stock and 42 % of them had antibiotic stocks (21). Higgins, Wainright, Lu and Carrico (2004), in their study on 116 hospitals in Kentucky, found that the isolation and decontamination abilities of hospitals were insufficient in cases of mass injury (22).

It has been determined in the majority of hospitals where data is collected within the provincial borders of Istanbul have hospital disasters plan. Aytekin (2003), in Istanbul Metropolitan Municipality within the boundaries of 50 private, 29 public in a total of 79 hospitals, including research shows that 65 % of hospitals have disaster plans (7). This situation shows that the rate of hospital with disaster plan within the provincial borders of Istanbul has increased and that the understanding of hospital disaster planning is more important than before. In the study conducted by İzmir Provincial Health Directorate and Emergency Medical Association (2008), it was determined that 76.2 % of the public and private hospitals out of 42 hospitals in İzmir have hospital disaster plans (23). According to Ersel, Aksay and Kıyan (2009) located in the department of emergency medicine at the university hospitals in Turkey, 53.5 % of the 28 university hospitals have determined that hospital disaster plan (24). The Turkish Medical Association (2009), in which the physicians work in the inpatient treatment institutions to evaluate the preparedness for unusual situations; 36.5 % of the 449 physicians who participated in the study reported that they had a hospital disaster plan, 16.7 % did not and 45.7 % stated that they did not know if there was a disaster plan in the hospital (25). Bozkırlı (2004), in his study on 31 hospitals in Ankara, found that 80.6 % of hospitals had a disaster plan (15). Balçık, Osmanoğlu, Sağlam and Özkan (2008), 7 hospitals in Ankara to assess the current situation in disaster management as a result of research; it was found that all of the hospitals had disaster plans, but the state of disaster preparedness was not sufficient (26). The number of hospital disaster plans varies from province to province and there is no hospital disaster plan in all hospitals; legal regulations on this issue are not known enough. In the study, since some of the hospitals that do not have a disaster plan stated that there is no disaster plan because it is not an obligatory and half of the hospitals that have a disaster plan stated that they did because of obligation. However, according to the Turkish health legislation, hospitals must have disaster plans. This shows that some of the hospitals do not fully know the legal obligations related to the disaster. Taviloglu, Yanar, Kavuncu, Ertekin and Guloglu (2005) conducted a research on the activities of the hospitals in the region after the terrorist bombings of 15 and

20 November 2003 in Istanbul. It was determined that 24 hospitals were involved in the first incident on November 15, 34 hospitals were involved in the second incident on November 20, 825 (330 and 495) patients were treated in hospitals and 144 (85 and 59) patients were hospitalized. At the end of this research, attention was paid to the fact that all hospitals have a disaster plan. It has been pointed out that losses can only be reduced by preparing these events in advance, planning, testing plans and training staff (27). Higgins et al. (2004), in their study on 116 hospitals in Kentucky; found that 99 % of the hospitals had a disaster plan (22). Remmen (2006) examined the preparation of the disaster plan of hospitals in the Netherlands in 1997–2002. In this study, the rate of hospital without a disaster plan was 7 % in 1997 and 1 % in 2002 (28).

It was found that two-fifths of the disaster plans of the hospitals were prepared specifically for the hospital, independent of the plans of other hospitals; it was determined that half of the hospitals were prepared by taking the plan prepared for another hospital and changing the characteristics of the hospital. As the disaster risk, facilities and capabilities of each hospital are different, the plan needs to be prepared in its own way.

In the vast majority of hospitals, the plan has been identified as a "Hospital Disaster Plan (HDP)", while in a few others it has been named under other names. Even though there are differences at the beginning of the plan even in the name of the plan, it shows that the standards are not determined and the common language cannot be provided. It is seen that also there is no common definition in the literature, similar topics were mentioned under the names of "Hospital Disaster Plan", "Hospital Emergency Plan", "Hospital Incident Plan" and "Emergency Management Plan". In a situation where many people from different disciplines work together, the use of common language and terminology is considered important.

In the half of the hospitals, in the period prior to the preparation of the plan, it was assumed that the senior management fully adopted the hospital disaster plan approach and fully supported the disaster plan at every stage during the plan preparation period. The lack of full adoption of the disaster plan approach by senior management shows that the plan is not exactly owned. As a matter of fact, only a quarter of the staff in the hospitals fully owned the plan. It would be difficult for an unfulfilled plan to succeed. The support and guidance of the senior management of the hospital should be seen as an indispensable condition of planning. Rüter, Nilsson and Vilkström (2006) compared the reactions of the management staff of 3 different hospitals in the disaster situation. Managers with low managerial abilities have also found that their staffing skills are also low (29).

In the period before the preparation of the plan, in order to prepare the plan in half of the hospitals, it was determined that the planning team was fully established and in one third of the preparatory program was prepared to prepare the plan. The lack of a program to prepare the plan and the establishment of a team show that some of the hospitals have not been fully prepared. However, it is thought that the success of the planning studies depends largely on the pre-planning preparations. According to Rivera and Char (2004), in the research of the hospitals in Louis-Missouri with 170 emergency services personnel, 16 % of the participants stated that the disaster planning team was not established and 23 % stated that there were no emergency service personnel in the team (30). Higgins et al. (2004), in their study on 116 hospitals in Kentucky; found that 95 % of the hospitals had a disaster planning committee (22).

In the plan preparation period; in only one fifth of the hospitals, it was determined that the vulnerability or risk analysis was fully performed and the strengths and weaknesses of the hospitals against disasters were determined precisely. The vulnerability and not conducting risk analysis indicates that the hazards that hospitals may be exposed have not been identified. It will not be possible to prepare for unknown dangers or the dangers that are not fully identified. As a matter of fact, in only one-fifth of hospitals, harm-reducing measures (structural reinforcement, etc.) were fully taken and non-structural hazards (fixing of devices, opening of exit paths, etc.) were fully reduced. Braun, Wineman, Finn, Barbera, Schmaltz and Loeb (2006) conducted research at 575 hospitals and found that 82.2 % of the hospitals conducted a vulnerability analysis (31).

In the plan preparation period, only one quarter of hospitals were fully coordinated with public and private institutions and organizations such as Health Directorate, Defense Directorate, Fire Brigade, 112, Police, etc. Also, it was determined that only one quarter of the hospitals provided delegation to the province/district disaster management activities and that the hospital disaster plan was fully compliant with the provincial/district regional/local disaster plans. This situation shows that the hospital disaster plans are mostly broken down from the external environment of the hospital and that there will be difficulties in the fulfillment of external environmental activities in case of a disaster. Niska and Burt (2005), in the United States in their research in 500 hospitals, three quarters of hospitals (76.4 %) found that they were included in local disaster plans (32). The disaster plans of the hospitals should be compatible with and approved by province health disaster and emergency plans.

Only a third of the hospitals had a full 24-hour contract with ambulance companies, air-conditioning technical services and medical consumables-pharmaceutical companies. Only one-tenth of the hospitals were found to have a full 24-hour contract with engineering institutions to assess the structural damage and safety of the hospital in the event of a disaster and with the health facilities to evacuate patients in case of a disaster. This condition shows that most hospitals that do not have contracts with the institutions will experience difficulties in meeting such services in the event of a disaster. Kaji and Lewis (2006), in their study on 45 hospitals, in the case of closure of the hospital in all of the hospitals have made agreements with various institutions and organizations (21).

More than half of the hospitals have been identified as a predetermined management chain to be deployed in the event of a disaster/incident and a predetermined management team has been fully established to serve in the event of a disaster. This shows that the majority of hospitals has adopted the Hospital Incident Command System approach and is ready to use a different management chain in case of a disaster. Chen and Wang (2005) examined the developmental impact of Hospital Emergency Incident Command System (HEICS) training on the practice. They compared the plans of the 51 emergency hospitals in Taipei one year ago and the performance of the plans after the HEICS training. A significant improvement was observed in 98 % of hospitals compared to the previous year. As a result, it is stated that HEICS training is critical to implementation (33).

It was determined that two thirds of the hospitals were fully determined by the person who will decide the partial or full evacuation in case of disasters. However, it was determined that only one third of the hospitals were determined exactly which health institutions the patients were to be discharged. This shows that in some of the hospitals, there is no adequate coordination with the external environment for evacuation and no evacuation protocols have been made.

Approximately one-fourth of the hospitals with disaster plan have been fully established in detail and the work plans and costing for the goals and targets are determined precisely by means of concrete and measurable objectives, targets, strategies, performance programs and activities and projects to be achieved in the medium term. This shows that the majority of hospitals do not adopt a strategic planning approach for disaster preparedness and that hospitals do not focus on the future of disaster preparedness, even though there is a disaster plan. Ginter, Duncan and Abdolrasulnia (2007) stated that hospitals should identify strategies for pre-disaster prevention and preparatory activities and post-disaster activities; for this reason, many hospitals have begun to preparation for disaster preparedness with strategic planning and have become a necessity (34).

In the period after the plan was prepared, it was determined that the feasibility of the plan was fully evaluated and updated in one-fifth of the hospitals which have disaster plan and disaster drills were conducted regularly. This situation shows that the majority of hospitals are made on paper due to various requirements and then abandoned to their fate. Heide (2007) stated that the fact that the hospital has a written plan does not mean that the hospital is ready for disaster (35). Of course the plan is important, but it is just one of the necessary conditions for preparation. If the other conditions are not fulfilled, the written plan will remain just a dream. In literature, this dream is called "the paper plan syndrome". Higgins et al. (2004), in their study on 116 hospitals in Kentucky; 81 % of hospitals have updated the disaster plan and 96 % of the annual disaster drills have been done (22). Thomas, Hsu, Kim, Colli, Arana and Green (2005) evaluated the disaster drills of a hospital. In this research, in order to identify the errors and deficiencies in the event management system, they stated that hospitals should be subjected to a structured, objective and measurable evaluation (36).

It is determined that there is no disaster management center located in approximately one-fifth of the hospitals which have and in a small part of the hospitals, this center can work for at least 1 week on a 24-hour basis without assistance. This situation shows that the understanding of disaster management center is not fully adopted by all hospitals.

Calculation and classification method, which is described in the section of materials and methods and calculated over 100 GENERAL scores; that two-fifths of the hospitals with a disaster plan have a good score and can be classified as a class A hospital for disaster planning; it was found that two out of five were rated as medium class and could be classified as a class B hospital for disaster planning and one-fifth were poorly rated and could be classified as a class C hospital for disaster planning (Tab. 7). According to the Hospital Safety Index, which is an example of classification; Class C hospitals need to complete their deficiencies in disaster planning urgently. Class B hospitals are still at risk for disaster planning and need to complete their deficiencies in the short term. In A class hospitals, disaster planning is sufficient in case of disaster but should continue to develop plans in medium and long term (13,14). In our study, the existence of a national institution which has been certifying hospitals in the presence of a national method for evaluating and measuring the disaster preparations of hospitals has not been established in our country. McCarthy, Brewster, Hsu, Macintyre and Kelen (2009) compared the practices of 5 different organizations (Veterans Health Administration, the Joint Commission, the Institute of Medicine, the Department of Homeland Security and the Department of Health and Human Services) in the United States on emergency management capabilities of health facilities in the United States. In this study, they determined that there is no widely accepted, approved system to guide health facilities in disaster preparedness and disaster-related activities. Although some organizations have tools for evaluating health facilities, they are not fully tested for their reliability and validity (37). Adini, Goldberg, Cohen and Bar-Dayan (2008) used a tool created by specialists to assess the quality of standard operating procedures that hospitals prepare for pandemic influenza. With this 31-item instrument, the pandemic influenza standard operating procedures of 24 hospitals in Israel were evaluated under 7 headings. At the end of the study, it was determined that only 2 of the 7 measurements were reliable and 2 measurements did not provide sufficient correlation. It was stated that the measurement method developed at the end of the study could be a model for the evaluation process of the hospitals, although not high reliability (38). Kaji and Lewis (2008) tested the reliability of the Johns Hopkins University AHRQ (Agency for Healthcare Research and Quality) hospital disaster assessment tool in 6 hospitals. In this study, the reliability of the assessment tool has found well. In this study, 4 hours of education was used. They have concluded that the assessment tool should be used after adequate training is given to the auditors, because some students have reached different measurements on the same subject (39). Oster and Chaffee (2004) examined the emergency preparedness of 34 hospitals with the Hospital Emergency Analysis Tool (HEAT), which they prepared using 240 critical preparatory factors. It has been emphasized that the prepared analysis tool can be used to determine the strengths and weaknesses of hospitals and that hospitals should strictly supervise emergency preparedness (40).

It was determined that the HDP scores of non-ERH were higher than those of state hospitals. The rate of ERH was found to be high among state hospitals identified as class C with HDP point, while the rate of hospitals with non-ERH was higher among state hospitals identified as Class A (Tab. 8). This shows that the preparation of non-ERH is better than ERH. Comparisons according to the amount of beds also support this finding. It is predicted that the hospitals with more than 400 beds (most of them are ERH) are low compared to hospitals with less than 400 beds. The reasons for this difference in ERH may need to be investigated in more detail.

All scores of hospitals with JCI accreditation were found to be significantly higher than the scores of hospitals without JCI accreditation. In HDP and GENERAL scoring, the rate of having JCI accreditation is high among hospitals which are considered to be A class (Tab. 10). This condition indicates that JCI accreditation has a positive effect on the disaster/emergency preparedness of hospitals. Jenkins, Kelen, Sauer, Fredericksen and McCarthy (2009) compared the compliance of 9 different hospital emergency preparedness assessment tools with the National Incident Management System (NIMS) guidelines. In this study, they found that vehicles could not establish a standard in terms of compliance with NIMS rules evaluation tools were scored under 4 headings and the highest three scores were obtained by VHA (Veterinary Health Administration), TJC (The Joint Commission) and APIC (Association for Professionals in Infection Control and Epidemiology) assessment tools, respectively. The need to re-examine and update assessment tools is emphasized (41). Niska and Burt (2006) determined that hospital staff (doctor, nurse, laboratory assistant) accredited by the Joint Commission received training on preparing terrorism higher than other hospitals (42).

Conclusion

As a result, although the majority of hospitals (87 %) had a hospital disaster plan, it was determined that hospitals did not fully perform the activities in the disaster planning process at the same rate. When the facilities and capabilities of the hospitals are examined, the same rate of competence has not been determined. The developed scoring method supported this finding and only two-fifths of the hospitals were found to have sufficient disaster planning activities. Thus, the high rate of being a hospital disaster plan should not be deceptive. The fact that having the disaster plan does not mean that the hospital is ready for disaster is fully supported by the literature. With the data collection tool developed, the general situation analysis of the disaster planning activities of the hospitals in Istanbul was conducted, which resources are currently available or which aspects are lacking, positive or negative developments beyond the control of the hospital have been evaluated.

The fact that hospitals have disaster plans does not necessarily mean that they are ready for disaster is a necessity to evaluate and measure the disaster planning of hospitals. Even in this case, it is seen that a scale or a tool is needed to make the evaluation. With this research, a scale/tool was developed to evaluate the disaster planning of hospitals. Of course, this scale can be improved to be more comprehensive. However, the scale is considered to be an example in the evaluation of disaster planning of hospitals.

In order to complete disaster preparedness of hospital, future goals and objectives should be defined and then these methods and objectives should be determined. This situation shows that strategic planning approach can be used in disaster planning of hospitals.

In Turkey, a document of guidance for hospitals to do their disaster preparedness was published in 2015 (43). There is a requirement for a national system to evaluate, measure and certify the disaster preparedness of hospitals. It is appropriate to evaluate, measure, drill and ultimately certify plans with unknown validity and reliability. Of course, the personnel should be included in this system should also have the competency to evaluate the preparedness of the hospitals. It is evaluated that disaster preparedness status of a hospitals can only be determined by a committee of representatives from different disciplines such as building engineers, architects trained in hospital design, medical–non-medical device specialists, medical staff (doctor, nurse), logistics/administrative staff, security personnel etc.

References

1. Krajewski MJ, Sztajnkrycer M, Báez AA. (2005). Hospital Disaster Preparedness in the United States: New Issues, New Challenges. *The Internet Journal of Rescue and Disaster Medicine*, Vol. 4, Number 2.

2. Sur H. (2005). Hastane Afet Planı. In: *Sağlık İşletmelerinde Yönetim*. Eds: Hayran O, Sur H, SAYED Yayınları, p.57–76.

3. Tarakcıoğlu H, Atilla R, Ersoy G, Aktepe T, Sarıoğlu S. (2002). Hastane Olağandışı Durum Sistemi. In: 5. *Ulusal Sağlık Kuruluşları ve Hastane Yönetimi Sempozyumu Bildiriler Kitabı*. Eskişehir, p.122–127.

4. Pan American Health Organization Regional Office of the World Health Organization. (2000). Principles of Disaster Mitigation in Health Facilities.

5. Yarar O. (2005). Afetlerde Hastane ve Hastane Yönetim Hizmetleri. In: *Afet Tıbbı*. Eds: Eryılmaz M, Dizer U, Ünsal Yayınları, Ankara, p.635–640.

6. Hersche B, Wenker OC. (2000). Principles of Hospital Disaster Planning. *The Internet Journal of Rescue and Disaster Medicine*, Volume 1, Number 2.

7. Aytekin T. (2003). İstanbul Büyükşehir Belediyesi Sınırları İçinde Yer Alan Hastanelerde Afet Yönetimine İlişkin Mevcut Durumun Değerlendirilmesi. Marmara Üniversitesi Sağlık Bilimleri Enstitüsü, Yüksek Lisans Tezi, İstanbul, (Danışman: Yrd. Doç. Dr. S Kalaça).

8. Koçel T. (2005). İşletme Yöneticiliği. Arıkan Basım Yayım Dağıtım Ltd. Şti., 10.Bası, Denizli.

9. T.C. Kalkınma Bakanlığı. (2018). Kamu İdareleri İçin Stratejik Planlama Kılavuzu, 3. Sürüm.

10. Rodoplu Ü, Ersoy G. (2005). Hastane Afet Planı. In: *Afet Tıbbı*. Eds: Eryılmaz M, Dizer U, Ünsal Yayınları, Ankara, p.619–625.

11. Altıntop İ. (2006). Erciyes Üniversitesi Tıp Fakültesi Hastaneleri Afet Planı. Erciyes Üniversitesi Tıp Fakültesi, Tıpta Uzmanlık Tezi, Kayseri, (Danışman: Doç. Dr. İ İkizceli).

12. Eli Lilly National Clinical Audit Centre. (1996). A Method for Surveying Patient Satisfaction, Instructions for Audit Groups. University of Leicester, Leicester.

13. World Health Organization. (2015) . Hospital Safety Index: Guide For Evaluators, 2nd ed..

14. Pan American Health Organization Regional Office of the World Health Organization. (2008). Evaluation Forms for Safe Hospitals.

15. Bozkırlı K. (2004). Afet ve Felaketlerde Hastane Hizmetlerinin Yönetimi: Bir Alan Çalışması. Gazi Üniversitesi Sosyal Bilimler Enstitüsü, Yüksek Lisans Tezi, Ankara, (Danışman: Doç. Dr. D Tengilimoğlu).

16. Bartley BH, Stella JB, Walsh LD. (2006). What a Disaster?! Assessing Utility of Simulated Disaster Exercise and Associated Educational Process. *Prehospital and Disaster Medicine*, 21(4):249–255.

17. Sarp N, İşlek E. (2006). Hastane Personelinin Yangın Konusunda Bilgi Düzeyinin Saptanması. *Ulusal Afet Dergisi*, Cilt 1, Sayı 1.

18. Paul JA, Lin L. (2009). Impact of Facility Damages on Hospital Capacities for Decision Support in Disaster Response Planning for an Earthquake. *Prehospital and Disaster Medicine*, 24(4):333–341.

19. İstanbul Büyükşehir Belediyesi Planlama ve İmar Dairesi Zemin ve Deprem İnceleme Müdürlüğü. (2003). İstanbul İçin Deprem Master Planı.

20. American College of Emergency Physicians, Federal Emergency Management Agency (FEMA). (2005). Community Healtcare Disaster Preparedness Assessment Survey.

21. Kaji AH, Lewis RJ. (2006). Hospital Disaster Preparedness in Los Angeles County. *Academic Emergency Medicine*, 13:1198–1203.

22. Higgins W, Wainright C, Lu N, Carrico R. (2004). Assessing Hospital Preparedness Using an Instrument Based on the Mass Casualty Disaster Plan Checklist: Results of a Statewide Survey. *American Journal of Infection Control*, 32:327–332.

23. İzmir İl Sağlık Müdürlüğü, Türkiye Acil Tıp Derneği. (2008). İzmir İli Sağlık Hizmetleri Afetlere Hazırlık Programı. Hastane Afet Planlaması Ön Değerlendirme Anketi Çalışması.

24. Ersel M, Aksay E, Kıyan S. (2009). Türkiye'deki acil tıp anabilim dallarının afetlere hazırlık ve eğitim düzeyleri. *Türkiye Acil Tıp Dergisi*, Cilt:9, Sayı:3, p.115–121.

25 .Türk Tabipleri Birliği. (2009). Hekimlerin Çalıştıkları Yataklı Tedavi Kurumlarının Olağandışı Durumlara Yönelik Hazırlıklılığını Değerlendirmeleri Araştırması.

26. Balçık PY, Osmanoğlu MA, Sağlam Ö, Özkan MH. (2008). Ankara'da seçilen bazı hastanelerde afet yönetimine ilişkin mevcut durumun değerlendirilmesi. *Sağlık İdarecileri Derneği, Sağlık ve Hastane İdaresi Kongresi, Uluslararası Katılımlı, Bildiriler Kitabı*, Eds: Esatoğlu AE, Ak B,

22–26 Ekim 2008, Queen's Park Resort Otel Tekirova-Kemer/Antalya, p.250–259.

27. Taviloglu K,Yanar H, Kavuncu A, Ertekin C, Guloglu R. (2005). 2003 Terrorist Bombings in Istanbul. *International Journal of Disaster Medicine*, 1–4: 45–49.

28. Remmen JV. (2006). The Status of the Hospital Disaster Plan in the Netherlands. *International Journal of Disaster Medicine*, 3(1): 28–31.

29. Rüter A, Nilsson H, Vilkström T. (2006). Performance Indicators as Quality Control for Testing and Evaluating Hospital Management Groups: A Pilot Study. *Prehospital and Disaster Medicine*, 21(6): 423–426.

30. Rivera AF, Char DM. (2004). Emergency Department Disaster Preparedness: Identifying the Barriers. *Annals of Emergency Medicine*, 44(4) (Suppl):p.94.

31. Braun BI, Wineman NV, Finn NL, Barbera JA, Schmaltz SP, Loeb JM. (2006). Integrating Hospitals into Community Emergency Preparedness Planning. *Annals of Internal Medicine*, 144: 799–811.

32. Niska RW, Burt CW. (2005). Bioterrorism and Mass Casualty Preparedness in Hospitals: United States, 2003. *Advance Data from Vital and Health Statistics*, Number 364.

33. Chen HT, Wang TL. (2005). Impact of Hospital Emergency Incident Command System (HEICS) Training on Disaster Preparedness of Emergency Response Hospitals. *Annals of Disaster Medicine*, 4: 7–11.

34. Ginter PM, Duncan WJ, Abdolrasulnia M. (2007). Hospital Strategic Preparedness Planning: The New Imperative. *Prehospital and Disaster Medicine*, 22 (6): 529–536.

35. Heide EAD. (2007). Principles of Hospital Disaster Planning. In: *Disaster Medicine*. Eds: Hogan DE, Burstein JL, 2nd ed, Lippincott Williams & Wilkins, p. 95–126.

36. Thomas TL, Hsu EB, Kim HK, Colli S, Arana G, Green GB. (2005). The Incident Command System in Disasters: Evaluation Methods for a Hospital-Based Exercise. *Prehospital and Disaster Medicine*, 20 (1):14–23.

37. McCarthy ML, Brewster P, Hsu EB, Macintyre AG, Kelen GD. (2009). Consensus and Tools Needed to Measure Health Care Emergency Management Capabilities. *Disaster Medicine and Public Health Preparedness*, 3 (1): 45–51.

38. Adini B, Goldberg A, Cohen R, Bar-Dayan B. (2008). Relationship between Standards of Procedures for Pandemic Flu and Level of Hospital Performance in Simulated Drills. *Annals of Emergency Medicine*, 52: 223–229.

39. Kaji AH, Lewis RJ. (2008). Assessment of the Reliability of the Johns Hopkins/Agency for Healthcare Research and Quality Hospital Disaster Drill Evaluation Tool. *Annals of Emergency Medicine*, 52: 204–210.

40. Oster NS, Chaffee MW. (2004). Hospital Preparedness Analysis Using the Hospital Emergency Analysis Tool (The HEAT). *Annals of Emergency Medicine*, 44(4)(Suppl):p.61.

41. Jenkins JL, Kelen GD, Sauer LM, Fredericksen KA, McCarthy ML. (2009). Review of Hospital Preparedness Instruments for National Incident Management System Compliance. *Disaster Medicine and Public Health Preparedness*, 3(Suppl):p. 83–89.

42. Niska RW, Burt CW. (2006). Training for Terrorism-Related Conditions in Hospitals: United States, 2003–04. *Advance Data from Vital and Health Statistics*, Number 380.

43. T.C. Sağlık Bakanlığı. (2015). Hastane Afet ve Acil Durum Planı (HAP) Hazırlama Kılavuzu.

List of Figures

List of Tables

About the Editor

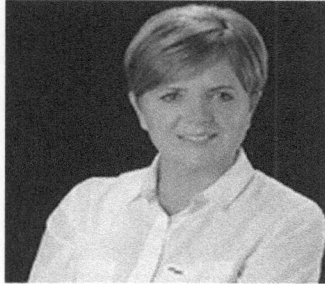

Prof. Dr. Fatma Eti Aslan
Dean of Faculty of Health Sciences at Bahcesehir Universityi, Istanbul, Turkey
Professor Eti Aslan obtained her nursing license from the Istanbul University Florence Nightingale Nursing School in 1986, her master degree from Istanbul University Institute of Health Sciences Department of Nursing in 1988, her doctoral degree from Istanbul University Institute of Health Sciences Department of Medical Surgical Nursing in 1992. She worked at Cerrahpasa Hospital as a nurse for three years and then at Marmara University as an assistant professor between 1993–1999, as an associate professor between 1999–2006 and as a professor between 2006–2009. She is still working at Bahcesehir University Faculty of Health Sciences as a head of Nursing program and as a dean of faculty. Professor Eti Aslan managed 43 master's thesis and four (4) doctorate thesis until now. She is an author of four (4) nursing books, editor of 12 books, author of lots of chapters and she also has 34 international SCI, SSCI scientific papers, 98 national papers and 53 international congress participation. She continues to teach continuously.

******

The increased knowledge in health care and the development of healthcare technologies is a great contribution to scientific studies in this field. In this context, the book will contribute to the development of health sciences and the quality of patient care in a total of 14 scientific original research article of which eight on physiotherapy and rehabilitation, five on nursing, and one on health management. A total of 29 researchers/writers who contributed to these research articles prepared with great labour and scientific meticulously, and also for their contributions in the selection of articles and the preparation of the book for publication, I would like to thank Hayat Yalın, Hasan Kerem Alptekin, İshak Aydemir for their contributions to the health sciences and Fadime Çınar for editorial support.

www.ingramcontent.com/pod-product-compliance
Lightning Source LLC
Chambersburg PA
CBHW020834210326
41598CB00019B/1899